## 1    Introduction

**D**arwin's proposition that all species of life have descended over time from common ancestors is now widely accepted and considered a foundational concept in science. He describes how all living things develop in the face of survival pressures and opportunities by adapting and changing. Since Darwin's original published work, "On the Origin of Species," in 1859, many advances have been made. Archaeology, with its extended view of this planet's fossil evidence, shows how over long periods of time animals and plants change. Darwin's finches who live on different islands in the Galapagos have developed different beak shapes and strategies for feeding according to the island where they live.

After physical death, and the soul moves through different Bardo states, the soul's Karma determines how the soul will be reincarnated. Helping the soul through the different states may be aided by a Shaman.

In this book we look at evolution and how it affects physical form, and how Karma resulting from life experience affects the soul and its reincarnation. Both are intimately linked, and both take time, a lot of time, things do not happen overnight. The soul is reborn into a physical body, a container for it, while it harvests lessons and karma from a lifetime of existence. Both the physical container and the soul are increasingly subject to human intervention, which we will look at.

This book is part of a series which includes broad introductions into shamans and shamanism. This book concentrates on reincarnation and the beliefs and rituals that surround the soul. This book is connected to an episode of The Shaman Podcast.

The Reiki, Shamanism and the essential loving mysticism is complementary to our:

- YouTube video series, "Reiki and Shamanism,"

- "The Shaman Podcast" on iTunes, Spotify, Google Podcasts, iHeart Radio, Stitcher, Tunine, Deezer and more.

Connect with our Private Facebook group to learn more about Reiki.

Subscribe to our newsletter to learn more about Reiki and Shamanism.

Enjoy.                                                  https://www.markaashford.com
Mark Ashford, MSc,                          Information@markaashford.com
Usui Tibetan Reiki Master and Teacher

Evolution and Karma

## 2 Table of contents

1 Introduction....................................................................................................1

2 Table of contents ...........................................................................................3

3 Table of figures .............................................................................................6

4 Charles Darwin...............................................................................................7

4.1 Etymology—Atheism......................................................................7

5 Evolution—Darwinism ....................................................................................9

5.1 Competition:.................................................................................9

5.2 Heritable Differences:....................................................................9

5.3 Survival of the Fittest:...................................................................9

5.4 Descent with Modification/Phylogenesis: .........................................9

5.5 In Summary ................................................................................10

5.6 Evolution cannot Create Perfection. ...............................................10

5.7 Good Enough Is Good Enough .......................................................10

5.8 Complexity of Evolution................................................................11

6 Processes of Evolution ..................................................................................12

6.1 Mutation ....................................................................................12

6.2 Sex and Genetic Stuffing .............................................................12

6.3 Migration....................................................................................13

6.4 Genetics ....................................................................................13

6.5 Genetic Drift...............................................................................14

6.6 Natural Selection.........................................................................14

6.7 Species Development ...................................................................14

6.8 Gradual Versus Rapid Change .......................................................15

6.9 Adaptation .................................................................................15

6.10 Artificial Selection........................................................................16

6.11 Coevolution................................................................................16

7 Karma .........................................................................................................19

7.1 Description .................................................................................20

7.2 Parts of Karma............................................................................20

7.3 Karma is Not Fate .......................................................................22

8 Free Will ......................................................................................................23

8.1 Karma and Free Will.....................................................................23

8.2 Karmic Law.................................................................................25

9 Karma and Hinduism .....................................................................................26

10   Karma and Buddhism ....................................................................................................28

11   Karma in Tibetan Buddhism ........................................................................................30

12   Karma and Bon ..........................................................................................................30

13   Prayer Wheel—Chokhor..............................................................................................31

14   Karma and Jainism .....................................................................................................34

15   Karma and Sikhism .....................................................................................................35

16   Karma and Taoism ......................................................................................................36

17   Karma and Orthodox Christianity ................................................................................37

18   Karma and Catholicism ...............................................................................................38

19   Karma and Islam .........................................................................................................40

20   Karma and Protestantism............................................................................................41

22   Karma in the West ......................................................................................................42

23   Karma in New Age ......................................................................................................43

24   Karma in Science .......................................................................................................45

25   Karma Fruit Bearing or the Result..............................................................................46

26   Karmic Accumulation and Debt ..................................................................................47

27   What is the Soul? .......................................................................................................49

27.1     Etymology...........................................................................................................49

27.2     A Definition ........................................................................................................49

27.3     Dictionary Definition ..........................................................................................49

27.4     Atman—Hinduism..............................................................................................50

27.5     Theological Soul ................................................................................................50

27.6     Where Is the Soul in the Physical Body? ..........................................................52

27.7     Ensoulment.......................................................................................................52

27.8     Shamanic Soul..................................................................................................53

28   Rebirth .......................................................................................................................55

28.1     Is Rebirth Simultaneous? .................................................................................55

28.2     Reaching Rebirth ..............................................................................................56

29   Mindfulness................................................................................................................58

30   Bardo..........................................................................................................................61

30.1     Bardo States.....................................................................................................63

30.2     The Six Bardos in Tibetan Buddhism ...............................................................64

30.3     The Liberation Through Hearing During the Intermediate State...........................65

31   Karmic Evolution ...................................................................................68

32   Deafness.................................................................................................71

33   Darwin, Karma, and the Process of Rebirth...........................................75

33.1      Is Rebirth Simultaneous? ....................................................................75

33.2      Reaching Rebirth ..................................................................................76

33.3      Darwinian Evolution..............................................................................77

34   Differing Pace of Evolution and Karma.................................................80

35   Bibliography ...........................................................................................82

## 3    Table of figures

Figure 1. Karma. Photo by Levi XU on Unsplash ...................................................................18
Figure 2. Large Prayer Wheels at a Monastery ....................................................................33
Figure 3. Rebirth. Photo by kaleb tapp on Unsplash ...........................................................54
Figure 4. Be Mindful. Photo by Lesly Juarez on Unsplash ..................................................58
Figure 5. Be mindful.............................................................................................................58
Figure 6. Meditating in Nature. Photo by Steven Cordes on Unsplash................................60
Figure 7. Looking at Evolution..............................................................................................67
Figure 8. Help. Photo by J W on Unsplash...........................................................................70
Figure 9. Table taken from "Public address systems notify us of what's going on all the time, but a hearing-impaired individual probably won't get the message." ...........................................................................74

## 4    Charles Darwin

C harles Robert Darwin lived 73 years, from 12 February 1809 – 19 April 1882. His proposition that all species of life have descended over time from common ancestors is now widely accepted, and considered a foundational concept in science.[1]

Darwin's elegant vocabulary in his pivotal work, published in 1859, "On the Origin of Species" was disruptive for his time.

The Church of England's response was mixed. Darwin's old Cambridge tutors Sedgwick and Henslow dismissed the ideas, but liberal priests interpreted natural selection as an instrument of God's design, with the cleric Charles Kingsley seeing it as "just as noble a conception of Deity." In 1860, the publication of Essays and Reviews by seven liberal Anglican theologians diverted clerical attention from Darwin, with its ideas including higher criticism attacked by church authorities as heresy.[2]

As disruptive as it was, it was suitable for the level of academic knowledge and public and scientific appreciation of how species develop and change. It was limited by what we know today [2020] and also limited by the tools available to help Darwin gather and plan his theories, such as "Survival of the Fittest." We are, in all ways, consistent with the times in which we live. If you live in a time when there are no microscopes, you can only theorize about them, not see them.

To put it simply, Darwin travelled on a sailing ship, HMS Beagle, which relied on manually wound clocks, compasses, and sextant technology to identify its location. Today, we would use modern ships with GPS sensors and computers loaded with digital maps.
We have to consider the context of Darwin and his time as compared to ours. To what he had available to and what tools we have now.

The other point we need to recognize is that Darwin was ground breaking.

He was arriving at his theories, hypothesis and speaking up when the church was very much against him. Divine creation created all the things we see around us. There was no evolution, there was deliberate and considered thought, planning and execution of a plan by a divine being.

It was Darwin who had to deal with and suffer the debate between Science and Religion and the debate over the rise of Atheism, which appeared as part of the debate over science vs. religion. Atheism is, in the broadest sense, an absence of belief in the existence of deities. Less broadly, atheism is a rejection of the belief that any deities exist. In an even narrower sense, atheism is specifically the position that there are no deities. Atheism is contrasted with theism which in its most general form is the belief that at least one deity exists.[3]

### 4.1    Etymology—Atheism

---

[1] https://en.wikipedia.org/wiki/Charles_Darwin, "Charles Darwin."
[2] Ibid.
[3] Wikipedia, "Atheism."

The etymological root for the word atheism originated before the fifth century BCE from the ancient Greek atheos, meaning "without god(s)." In antiquity, it had multiple uses as a pejorative term applied to those thought to reject the gods worshiped by the larger society, those who were forsaken by the gods, or those who had no commitment to believe in the gods. The term denoted a social category created by orthodox religionists into which those who did not share their religious beliefs were placed. [4]

The actual term atheism emerged first in the 16th century. With the spread of free thought, skeptical inquiry, and subsequent increase in criticism of religion, the application of the term narrowed in scope. The first individuals to identify themselves using the word atheist lived in the 18th century during the Age of Enlightenment. The French Revolution, noted for its "unprecedented atheism", witnessed the first major political movement in history to advocate for the supremacy of human reason. [5]

---

[4] Ibid.
[5] Ibid.

## 5    Evolution—Darwinism

**D**arwinism is a theory of biological evolution developed by the English naturalist Charles Darwin (1809–1882) and others, stating that all species of organisms arise and develop through the natural selection of small, inherited variations that increase the individual's ability to compete, survive, and reproduce. Also called Darwinian theory, it originally included the broad concepts of transmutation of species or of evolution which gained general scientific acceptance after Darwin published On the Origin of Species in 1859, including concepts which predated Darwin's theories. English biologist Thomas Henry Huxley coined the term Darwinism in April 1860.[6]

The fundamental principles of Darwinism are below.

### 5.1    Competition:

In each species, each generation produces more individuals than can survive within their given environment. Individuals must then compete within their own species for natural resources, survival, and the chance to pass on their genes. This competition results in the survival of the fittest.

### 5.2    Heritable Differences:

Heritable differences can be found within the individuals of each species. These differences manifest themselves as visible and invisible traits and create advantages or disadvantages for the individual. From the perspective of a species, variation is preferred and necessary, as it provides a higher chance of survival for that species.

### 5.3    Survival of the Fittest:

The individuals with the genetic characteristics best suited for survival within the environment will survive and pass on their heritable genes. The advantages manifest themselves in many characteristics or traits—strength, speed, endurance, intelligence, social skills, resistance to pathogens, etc.

### 5.4    Descent with Modification/Phylogenesis:

The reproductive isolation of groups within a species leads to the diversion of genetic characteristics, which allows new species to emerge from a common ancestor. The line of descent from one common ancestor to the various species that have arisen is known as the Phylogenetic tree.

---

[6] Wikipedia, "Darwinism."

## 5.5    In Summary

Variation is a feature of natural populations and every population produces more progeny than its environment can manage. The consequences of this overproduction are that those individuals with the best genetic fitness for the environment will produce offspring that can more successfully compete in that environment. Thus, the subsequent generation will have a higher representation of these offspring and the population will have developed.  —Charles Darwin

## 5.6    Evolution cannot Create Perfection.

In the modern world, we are used to devices and things around us being "perfect" that are with no deficiencies that materially affect us. If things are imperfect when they go to market, they are redesigned, and the defects eliminated in future versions of the product or service.

A classic example we can all relate to is the evolution of the cell phone from the clumsy, heavy device with a massive battery to the slim, small, powerful devices we have today—2020.

Evolution of plants and animals, including humans, does not strive to create perfect versions of things. It is not following a design or design principles and does not value perfection over other valuable traits.

The fact is that evolution, as seen by Darwin, results from millennia of adaptation and change. Even with our abilities, human life is 100 years max, of which perhaps ¾ of that is useful and productive. We cannot see the changes that will take place in humanity in the next 100 years, let alone the next 1,000 years.

Because evolution is always, it can never go back and change mistakes and errors. A person with defective hearing would be susceptible to be attacked, robbed and killed because they could not hear their attacker. In 2020, we provide hearing aids that eliminate or at least reduce the deficiency in hearing. Weaknesses in human ability or "design," as long as they are not detrimental to survival, will always be with us.

The universe is so unhuman; it goes its way with so little thought of man. He is but an incident, not an end. We must adjust our notions to the discovery that things are not shaped to him, but that he is shaped by them. The air was not made for his lungs, but he had lungs because there was air; the light was not created for his eyes, but he has eyes because there is light. All the forces of nature are going their own way; man avails himself of them, or catches a ride as best he can. If he keeps his seat, he prospers; if he misses his hold and falls, he is crushed. *John Burroughs*[7]

## 5.7    Good Enough Is Good Enough

This principle speaks to the fact that "good enough" is all that is required for survival; being the fittest does not guarantee survival for the next generation. It also means that not all the evolutionary traits, good or bad, in the individual species member need to be perfect, just good enough of them. That is the goal of survival and evolution. We are not built or created to survive every situation existence throws at us. We just have to survive those that challenge us.

---

[7] "John Burroughs."

We consider that Good Enough is at the genetic level. Change happens at this level. Darwin's finches developed different beaks to allow them to feed according to the food that was available to them. The genes adapted and changed to create beaks that would allow its host animal to feed, breed, and survive. Every visible characteristic of humans, plants, and animals is derived from the DNA sequence in its cells.

## 5.8   Complexity of Evolution

Genetic changes are slight and incremental. As they grow and compound, the changes become more complex. Going back to Darwin's finches, the characteristics of their beaks speak to an evolutionary change driven by the need to feed and the food available to them on the islands they lived. Along with the differences in their beaks are differences in their inherited behaviour, which allows them to use their beaks effectively.

Evolution is not a genetically controlled distortion of one adult form into another; it is a genetically controlled alteration in a developmental program. —*Richard Dawkins*[8]

---

[8] "Richard Dawkins."

## 6    Processes of Evolution

**E**volution is the process by which modern organisms have descended from ancient ancestors. Evolution handles both the remarkable similarities we see across all life and the amazing diversity of that life.[9]

Fundamental to the process is a genetic variation upon which selective forces can act in order for evolution to occur..[10]

### 6.1    Mutation

Mutation is a driving force of evolution. It is a random change in an organism's genetic make-up, which influences the population's gene pool. It is a change in one or more chromosomes of the animal or plant's DNA. Mutations give rise to new alleles. An allele is—any of several forms of a gene, usually arising through mutation, that handle hereditary variation and source of genetic distinction in a population.

Mutations may be harmful or benign, but they are beneficial. For example, a mutation may permit organisms in a population to produce enzymes that will allow them to use certain food materials. Over time, these types of individuals survive, while those that don't have the mutations are more likely to perish.

Cells in our body contain DNA. There are lots of places for mutations to occur; however, not all mutations matter for evolution. Somatic mutations occur in non-reproductive cells and won't be passed onto offspring. For example, the golden colour on half of this Red Delicious apple was caused by a somatic mutation. The seeds of this apple do not carry the mutation. [11]

Mosoff the mutations that we think matter evolution are "naturally occurring." For example, when a cell divides, it makes a copy of its DNA—and sometimes the copy is not quite perfect. That slight difference from the original DNA sequence is a mutation.

Mutations can also be caused by exposure to specific chemicals or radiation. These agents cause the DNA to break down. This is not necessarily unnatural—even in the most isolated and pristine environments, DNA breaks down. When the cell repairs the DNA, it might not do a perfect job of the repair. So, the cell would end up with DNA slightly different from the original DNA and, hence, a mutation.[12]

For example, the golden colour on half of this Red Delicious apple was caused by a somatic mutation. The seeds of this apple do not carry the mutation. [13]

### 6.2    Sex and Genetic Stuffing

---

[9] https://evolution.berkeley.edu/evolibrary/article/evo_14, "Mechanisms the Processes of Evolution."
[10] Ibid.
[11] Ibid.
[12] Ibid.
[13] Ibid.

Sex can introduce new gene combinations into a population and is an important source of genetic variation. [14]

You probably know from experience that siblings are not genetically identical to their parents or to each other (except, of course, for identical twins). That's because when organisms reproduce sexually, some genetic "shuffling" occurs, bringing together new combinations of genes. For example, you might have bushy eyebrows and an enormous nose, since your mom had genes associated with bushy eyebrows and your dad had genes associated with an enormous nose. These combinations can be good, bad, or neutral. If your spouse is wild about the bushy eyebrows/big nose combination, you were lucky and hit on a winning combination! [15]

This shuffling is important for evolution because it can introduce new combinations of genes every generation. However, it can also break up "good" combinations of genes. [16]

Sexual selection is a "special case" of natural selection. Sexual selection acts on an organism's ability to get, often by any means necessary, or successfully copulate with a mate. [17]

Selection makes many organisms go to extreme lengths for sex. Some may be helpful but only for a limited period: the familiar brightly coloured fan developed by male peacocks requires maintenance and is a burden to them. It also advertises them to predators.

Animals who maintain either a territory for breeding or control of several females with which to breed require the male first fight and struggle to get the territory, or females, and then maintain them and breed with them. This is physically taxing and tiring. Fighting off other males who want territory or the females introduces the risk of injury.

The positive side to this approach is that the females can mate with males who are most able to produce good, fit young. So, both the male and female genes are passed forward into the next generation.

## 6.3    Migration

Some external factor either unable or forces a species to migrate to a new location. Usually, the external factor is resources, predominantly food. But climate can force migration, think in terms of ice ages, or extended periods of drought. Specialization of a species on a limited range of food sources that change and migrate, dragging those that feed on them with them.

## 6.4    Genetics

Another mechanism of evolution may occur during the migration of individuals from one group or location to another. When the migrating individuals interbreed with a new population, they contribute their genes to the gene pool of the local population. Maybe a superior gene in the

---

[14] Ibid.
[15] Ibid.
[16] Ibid.
[17] Ibid.

population existing in that location suppresses a gene of the population breeding itself into the local group. This establishes gene flow in the population.

Gene flow occurs, for example, when the wind carries seeds far beyond the bounds of the parent plant population. As another example, animals may be driven off from a herd by predators. Those animals form a new population, bringing new genes to a gene pool. Gene flow increases the similarity between remaining populations of the same species because it makes gene pools more similar to one another.

## 6.5   Genetic Drift

Imagine that in one generation, two brown beetles had four offspring each who survive to reproduce. Several green beetles were killed when predators fed on them and had no offspring. The next generation would have a greater number of brown beetles than the previous generation — but just by chance. These chance changes from generation to generation are known as genetic drift.

Another example of genetic drift, which can occur when a small group of individuals leaves a population and establishes a new one in a geographically isolated region. For example, when a small population of fish is placed in a lake, the fish population will develop into one that is different from the original. Fitness of a population is not considered genetic drift.

## 6.6   Natural Selection

Another mechanism for evolution is natural selection, which occurs when populations of organisms are subjected to the environment. The fittest creatures are more likely to survive and pass their genes to their offspring, producing a population that is better adapted to the environment. The genes of less fit individuals are less likely to be passed on to the next generation. The important selective force in natural selection is the environment.

Environmental fitness may be expressed in several ways. For example, it may involve an individual's ability to avoid predators, it may imply greater resistance to disease, it may enhance the ability to get food, or it may mean resistance to drought. Fitness may also be measured as enhanced reproductive ability, such as the ability to attract a mate. Better-adapted individuals produce relatively more offspring and pass on their genes more successfully than less-adapted individuals.

Several types of natural selection appear to affect populations. One type, stabilizing selection, occurs when the environment selects against organisms of a population with extreme versions of a trait. Another type of natural selection is disruptive selection. Here, the environment favours extreme types in a population at the expense of intermediate forms, splitting the population into two or more subpopulations. A third type of natural selection is directional selection. Here, the environment selects an extreme characteristic. The development of antibiotic-resistant bacteria in the modern era is an example of directional selection.

## 6.7   Species Development

A species is a group of individuals that share several features and can interbreed with one another, producing fertile offspring. When individuals of one species mate with individuals of a different species, any offspring are usually sterile. A species is also defined as a population whose members share a common gene pool.

The evolution of a species is speciation, which can occur when a population is isolated by geographic barriers, such as occurred in the isolation of Australia, New Zealand, and the Galapagos Islands. The variety of life forms found in Australia, but nowhere else, is an example of speciation by geographic barriers.

Speciation can also occur when reproductive barriers develop. For example, when members of a population develop anatomical barriers that make mating with other members of the population difficult, a new species can develop. The timing of sexual activity is another example of a reproductive barrier. Spatial difference, such as one species inhabiting treetops while another species lives at ground level, is another reason species develop.
Changes in the genes controlling development can have major effects on the morphology of the adult organism. Because these effects are so significant, scientists suspect that changes in developmental genes have helped bring about large-scale evolutionary transformations. Developmental changes may help explain, for example, how some hoofed mammals developed into ocean dwellers, how water plants invaded the land, and how small, armoured invertebrates developed wings.[18]

## 6.8    Gradual Versus Rapid Change

Darwin's theory included the observation that evolutionary changes take place slowly. Most times, the fossil record shows that a species changed gradually. The theory that evolution occurs gradually is known as gradualism.

In contrast to gradualism is the theory of punctuated equilibrium, which is a point of discussion among scientists. According to the theory of punctuated equilibrium, some species have long, stable periods of existence interrupted by relatively brief periods of rapid change.

Both groups of scientists agree that natural selection is the single most important factor in evolutionary changes in species. Whether the change is slow or punctuated and rapid, one thing is certain: Organisms have developed.

## 6.9    Adaptation

An adaptation is a feature that is common in a population because it provides some improved function. Adaptations are well fitted to their function and are produced by natural selection.

Adaptations can take many forms: a behaviour that allows better evasion of predators, a protein that functions better at body temperature, or an anatomical feature that allows the organism to access a valuable new resource—these might be adaptations. Many of the things that impress us most in nature are thought to be adaptations.

---

[18] Ibid.

For example, the creosote bush is a desert-dwelling plant that produces toxins that prevent other plants from growing nearby, thus reducing competition for nutrients and water.

Some adaptations are not helpful, such as vestigial structures. A vestigial structure is a feature that was an adaptation for the organism's ancestor, but that developed to be non-functional because the organism's environment changed. Fish species that live in completely dark caves have vestigial, non-functional eyes. When their sighted ancestors ended up living in caves, there was no longer any natural selection that maintained the function of the fishes' eyes. So, fish with better sight no longer outcompeted fish with worse sight. Today, these fishes still have eyes—but they are not functional and are not an adaptation; they are just the by-products of the fishes' evolutionary history.[19]

## 6.10  Artificial Selection

Long before Darwin and Wallace[20], farmers and breeders were using the idea of selection to cause major changes in the features of their plants and animals over decades. Farmers and breeders allowed only the plants and animals with desirable characteristics to reproduce, causing the evolution of farm stock. This process is called artificial selection because people, not nature, select which organisms get to reproduce. [21]

## 6.11  Coevolution

The term coevolution[22] is used to describe cases where two or more species reciprocally affect each other's evolution. So, for example, an evolutionary change in the morphology of a plant might affect the morphology of an herbivore that eats the plant, which might affect the evolution of the plant, which might affect the evolution of the herbivore and so on.

Coevolution is likely to happen when different species have close ecological interactions with one another. These ecological relationships include:

- Predator/prey and parasite/host

- Competitive species

- Mutualistic species

Plants and insects represent a classic case of coevolution—one that is often, but not always, mutualistic. Many plants and their pollinators are so reliant on one another and their relationships are so exclusive that biologists have good reason to think that the "match" between the two results from a coevolutionary process.

---

[19] Ibid.
[20] Wikipedia, "Alfred Russel Wallace."
[21] https://evolution.berkeley.edu/evolibrary/article/evo_14, "Mechanisms the Processes of Evolution."
[22] Wikipedia, "Coevolution."

But we can see exclusive "matches" between plants and insects even when pollination is not involved. Some Central American Acacia species have hollow thorns and pores at the bases of their leaves, that secret nectar. These hollow thorns are the exclusive nest site of some species of ant that drink the nectar. But the ants are not just taking advantage of the plant—they also defend their acacia plant against herbivores.

This system is probably the product of coevolution: the plants would not have developed hollow thorns or nectar pores unless their evolution had been affected by the ants, and the ants would not have developed herbivore defence behaviours unless their evolution had been affected by the plants.[23]

---

[23] https://evolution.berkeley.edu/evolibrary/article/evo_14, "Mechanisms the Processes of Evolution."

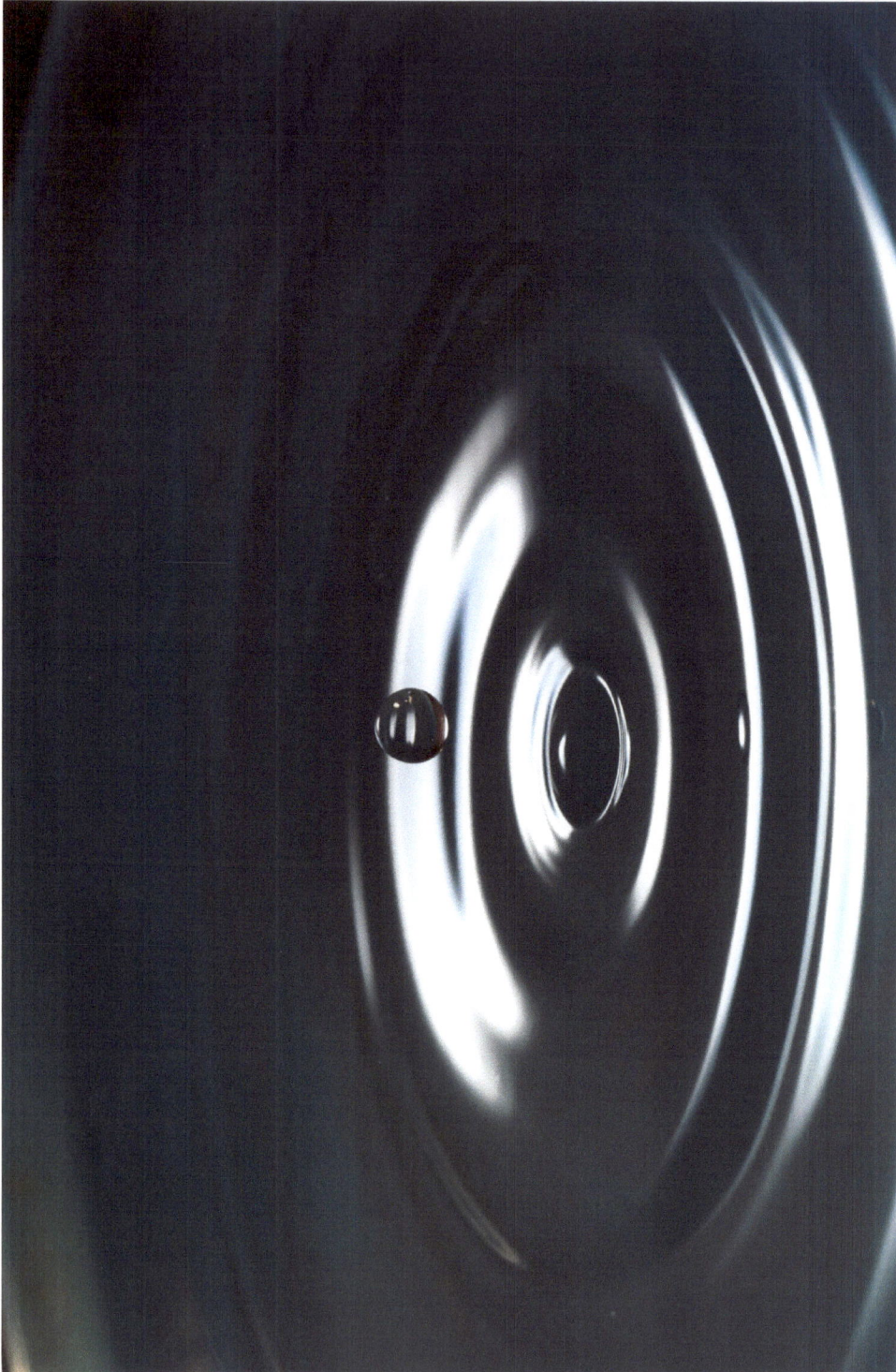

Figure 1. Karma. Photo by Levi XU on Unsplash

## 7    Karma

**K**arma comes from the Indian word Karmen. The Book of Mahabharata[24] is a major Sanskrit epic from ancient India. The book narrates the struggle between two groups of cousins, the Kaurava and the Pandava princes and their successors. The Kurukshetra War was fought between the two groups in Northern India, but the exact timing of it is open to conjecture. Current speculation is that the war marks the transition to Kaliyuga, which dates it to 3102 BCE.

The major battle is not the Mahabharata, but the fight between the gods Krishna[25] and Jarasandha[26], who is killed by Krishna. Ultimately, the Pandavas[27] and Balarama[28] take renunciation as Jain[29] monks and are reborn in heaven, while Krishna and Jarasandha are reborn in hell. In keeping with the law of karma, Krishna is reborn in hell for his exploits, sexual and violent excesses, while Jarasandha for his evil ways.

The Book of Mahabharata contains philosophical and devotional material, such as a discussion of the four "goals of life" or purusartha[30]. The word purusartha means human pursuit and refers to the four proper goals or aims of human life.

- Dharma[31] righteousness, moral values

- Artha[32] prosperity, economic values—at the personal level and society,

- Kama[33] pleasure, love, psychological values

- Moksha[34] liberation, spiritual value

In Indian literature, Dharma is emphasized in Artha and Kama; Moksha is the considered the goal of human life.

The philosophy of karma is closely associated with the idea of rebirth in many schools of Indian religions, particularly Hinduism[35], Buddhism[36], Jainism[37] and Sikhism[38] as well as Taoism[39]. In these schools, karma in the present affects one's future not just in what remains of your current life and

[24] Wikipedia, "Mahabharata."
[25] "Krishna."
[26] "Jarasandha."
[27] "Pandava."
[28] "Balarama."
[29] jainbelief.com, "Jainism."
[30] Wikipedia, "PuruṣāRtha."
[31] "Dharma."
[32] "Artha."
[33] "Kama."
[34] "Moksha."
[35] "Hinduism."
[36] "Buddhism."
[37] "Jainism."
[38] "Sikhism."
[39] "Taoism."

what you can do in it, but the nature and quality of future lives into which you are born—one's samsara.[40] [41]

## 7.1   Description

Karma operates through the law of cause and effect, action and reaction; it governs all life and binds the Atman[42] the Self, to the wheel of birth and death.

The process of action and reaction on all levels—physical and mental—is karma. God does not give us karma. We create our own. Karma is not fate; humans are believed to act with free will, creating their own destinies according to the Vedas,[43] a large body of religious texts originating in ancient India.

If an individual's goodness, he or she will reap goodness; if one sows evil, he or she will reap evil. Karma refers to the totality of humanity's actions and their associated reactions in current and previous lives, all of which determine the future. However, many karmas do not have an immediate effect; some accumulate and return unexpectedly in an individual's later lives. The conquest of karma is believed to lie in intelligent action and dispassionate reaction.[44]

## 7.2   Parts of Karma

Karma may be divided into different stages or parts regardless of whether karma is good or bad—table below:[45] [46]

| Karma | Description | Meaning |
|---|---|---|
| Sanchita karma[47] | accumulated actions | The sum of all karmas of this life and past lives. This is your store of karma. Think of karma like fruit. Not all apples on a tree mature on the same day, and it will be laden again in the next season and the next and so forth. It is for this reason that life is cyclical for an overwhelming majority of people. Why? If you plant apple trees, when the season comes, you will have plenty of apples. If you plant wild berries, however attractive, they are protected by thorny bushes, but like apples, they will flourish during their season. [48] |

---

[40] Ibid.

[41] https://en.wikipedia.org/wiki/Karma, "Karma."

[42] Wikipedia, "Atman."

[43] "Vedas."

[44] http://veda.wikidot.com/karma, "Karma Veda."

[45] Ibid.

[46] https://os.me/four-types-of-karma-explained-understanding-karma/, "4 Types of Karma - Understanding Karma in Spirituality."

[47] Wikipedia, "Sanchita Karma."

[48] https://os.me/four-types-of-karma-explained-understanding-karma/, "4 Types of Karma - Understanding Karma in Spirituality."

| Karma | Description | Meaning |
|---|---|---|
| Prarabdha karma[49] | Actions begun; set in motion | That portion of Sanchita[50] is karma that bears fruit and shapes the events and conditions of the current life, including one's body, and its personal tendencies and associations. Once you perform any karmic act, it is registered in the universe; it will come to fruition in due course. There is no escape. Whatever you are going through in life presently, note the word presently that you have no control over it, that is your *Prarabdha*.[51] |
| Kriyamana karma[52] | Being made | The karma being created and added to Sanchita[53] in this life by one's thoughts, words, and actions, or in the inner worlds between lives. The karma we are currently creating through our choices right now. It is our creativity that is unfolding; it is our "free will." |
| Agama karma[54] | Forthcoming, arriving, living, set in motion. | Are the actions that we are planning for the future actions that will or will not be achieved, depending on our choices, which are governed by our free will and which we are making now, and those that we have made in the past? The choices you make today have a direct bearing on your future tomorrow. What you do in the present moment determines what unfolds in the next. Agami karma is a mandatory karma. You have little choice, if any. If you have entered the orchard, perform the action of exciting as well, eventually.[55] |
| Vartamana Karma[56] | Present | Your fulfillment will not come from becoming someone other than yourself and being true to yourself by creating your own home. However, welcome you may be in another home; however hospitable your host may be, a while later, you no longer feel at home. You only feel at home in your own home. You may have ideals or idols, but it is important to be yourself, to discover yourself and your own truth. [57] |

[49] Ibid.

[50] Wikipedia, "Sanchita Karma."

[51] https://os.me/four-types-of-karma-explained-understanding-karma/, "4 Types of Karma - Understanding Karma in Spirituality."

[52] Wikipedia, "Kriyamana Karma."

[53] "Sanchita Karma."

[54] https://os.me/four-types-of-karma-explained-understanding-karma/, "4 Types of Karma - Understanding Karma in Spirituality."

[55] Ibid.

[56] Ibid.

[57] Ibid.

## 7.3 Karma is Not Fate

Karma has suffered a chronic miss association with the word fate or destiny.

Fate is a Western idea, derived largely from the three Abrahamic religions: Judaism, Christianity, and Islam. It means, with wide variation, that one's life has been set by agencies outside oneself, and as a result, we are helpless to change anything in it. We simply go from birth to death with a belief that something is supposed to be happening as decided by a power, outside of ourselves and which is greater than ourselves.

Fate/destiny cannot be understood by people. Because a greater power is involved in setting one's fate or destiny, so what is to come next in our lives is beyond human comprehension. Fate is so powerful it controls the outcome of a person's life before it happens. Many people become victims of fate and devote a lot of effort, time, and money into discovering what their fate or destiny is. They are absorbed in what will happen next in their lives and pay less attention to the effort, choices, and decisions they are making.

Karma is exactly the opposite.[58]

---

[58] http://veda.wikidot.com/karma, "Karma Veda."

## 8   Free Will

W hen we think about free will, we have to also think of some limitations that apply to it. Three limitations appear:

- Absolute Free will

Interesting, but there are things we cannot perform, no matter how much we want to. No matter how much we believe in absolute free will, we cannot make them happen.

As a scuba diver, I learned that as much as I would like to, I cannot breathe underwater, from the water, in the way fish do. I have to wear heavy scuba gear, and that the tank on my back contains a finite amount of air, which limits the time I can be underwater.

Besides the physical restraint of needing to breathe air, there is the mental or psychological issue of being underwater and breathing. The mechanics of breathing through my mouth and *never* through my nose were one thing, but as I sat on the bottom of the deep end of the swimming pool for the first time, I looked up and watched my class mates thrashing around on the surface, some having *intense* problems with what I found easy and even calming, though I had experienced nothing like it before.

I have described scuba diving to many people. Some are fascinated; most are fearful or express abhorrence at trying it. To them, the skills and requirements of diving are constraints that stop them and they have no control over them, nor do they wish to challenge blocks.

- No Free Will

While most people believe we freely choose our actions, they also accept we are free to resist impulses such as experiencing diving. Consciously or not, many people accept they are not meant, or able, to learn the intricacies and rules of scuba diving. They take a fatalistic approach to this limitation on their experiences.

According to fatalism, we cannot choose to do anything. Everything we do is predestined, and our feeling of being free to choose something other than what is preordained is an illusion. Fatalism is impossible to prove, but it's also impossible to disprove because a fatalist would say that whatever we do or say to disprove fatalism is itself determined by fate![59]

- Limited Free Will

  While I may not breathe underwater like a fish, I have enough free will to learn the skills and understand the equipment that will allow me, for a limited time, to exist underwater. That limited amount of free will includes what is necessary to challenge my mental and psychological prohibitions against opening my mouth and trying to breathe underwater.

### 8.1   Karma and Free Will

---

[59] David Pratt, "Fate or Free Will?."

Karma works to develop our ability to handle free will responsibly. [60]

Karma operates impersonally, giving us the opportunity at every moment to become open to greater levels of love and compassion through our experiences. The goal is to give us the experiences we need to strengthen into greater levels of awareness and responsibility. What we do at every moment is our choice. Once we accept total responsibility for who we are, for what we have done or will do, and for all our choices, life straightens out. [61]

The choices we make are influenced by the habitual patterns of thought, feeling, and behaviour arising from our past. From the moment we are born, we begin to display certain distinctive character traits, which are then developed or changed in the course of our lives as we react to circumstances and interact with people around us—partly passively, partly instinctually, and partly actively or self-consciously. But where does our basic character come from? There are three answers to this question.[62]

- Materialists would argue our basic character is determined by the genes we inherit from our parents, and by which of these genes are activated in our bodies. If asked why we have the parents we do have, and what determines which genes are active and which are recessive, they would answer in a single word: chance. But invoking chance explains nothing; it implies, in fact, that there is no explanation: things are the way they are. Efforts to reduce the wonders of life and mind to random phase-chemical interactions are grossly inadequate and unsatisfactory. [63]

- God, a divine being, who creates a new human soul for each newborn child. If God gives us our character and decides the circumstances of our birth, he would also bear a major responsibility for all the subsequent events of our lives. It would mean that people suffer because it's God's will that they should suffer. A being capable of such cruelty and injustice would surely be a senseless fiend rather than a "god." An extreme version of this position can be found in the Presbyterian Westminster Confession of Faith (3.6.016), which states: "By the decree of God, for the manifestation of his glory, some men and angels are predestinated unto everlasting life and others foreordained to everlasting death." Hardly an inspiring doctrine! [64]

- Reincarnation. The most reasonable. According to this view, our souls are reborn on earth again and again, and in each life, we reap what we have sown in previous lives and sow seeds we shall harvest in future lives. There is no such thing as chance, but a web of cause and effect, or karma, whereby the consequences of all our thoughts and deeds ultimately rebound upon ourselves, either in this life or in a future life. When a soul returns to incarnation, it is drawn by an affinity to the parents who can provide it with the body and

---

[60] http://veda.wikidot.com/karma, "Karma Veda."
[61] Ibid.
[62] Pratt, "Fate or Free Will?."
[63] Ibid.
[64] Ibid.

environment best fitted to the tendencies it already possesses. So rather than inheriting our characteristics from our parents, we actually inherit them through our parents from ourselves—from our own past. [65]

## 8.2   Karmic Law

In this book, we often talk about good and bad karma and in the west especially, there is a concept of an accounting, like balance sheet, and Excel worksheet if you like, with a row for each one of our good or bad karmic actions recorded in it. One column for Good Karma, one column for Bad Karma. At the bottom of the worksheet, the columns are totalled and a net or balance of karma is created. If the balance is positive, i.e., the good karma you have accumulated outweighs the bad karma, your rebirth will be favourable. If the opposite is true, rebirth will be unfavourable.

Karmic law does not provide for "netting out" good and bad karmic events. It is the <u>consequences</u> of Good and Bad karmic actions that our soul is here to *experience* and which are important learning exercises for our soul. The key word is "learning." Learning from the consequences of good karmic actions and from bad is the key message here. Good karmic actions give rise to pleasant experiences and consequences. Bad karmic actions give rise to unpleasant experiences and consequences.

A significantly good karmic action will not diminish an offensive action. For example, gifting a wheelchair to someone who cannot walk does not diminish the karmic consequences of harming another person. Each is separate; the consequences and understandings of each must be experienced separately.

Karma cannot be valued. You cannot make a charitable donation and say that good karma from the donation is worth $10 because no value can be attached to the pleasant experiences you will receive because of the donation. If you insult someone, you cannot say that negative karma is worth $5. Again, learning from the consequences and results of good and bad karmic actions are the key messages.

The soul of the person is not bound or part of what gives rise to Karma. It is the ego, which has been created through false impositions that bind karma, and it is the ego that experiences the fruits of karma.

---

[65] Ibid.

## 9   Karma and Hinduism

**H**induism is the major religion of India, practised by over 80% of the population. In 2020, the Indian population is projected to be 1.38 billion. In contrast to other religions, it has no founder. It is considered being the oldest religion in the world; it dates back to prehistoric times.[66]

No single creed or doctrine binds Hindus together. Intellectually there is complete freedom of belief, and one can be a monotheist[67], polytheist[68], or atheist[69]. Hinduism is a syncretic religion, welcoming and incorporating a variety of outside influences.[70]

The most ancient sacred texts of the Hindu religion are written in Sanskrit and are called the Vedas (vedah means "knowledge"). There are four Vedic books, of which the Rig-Veda is the oldest. It discusses multiple gods, the universe, and creation. The dates of these works are unknown. Many present-day Hindus rarely refer to these texts, but venerate them.

Hinduism accepts the concept of reincarnation. All living organisms, whether they are plants or gods, are caught in a cosmic cycle of birth, death, and rebirth. This cycle is repeated repeatedly. Life is determined by the law of karma.

Karma, in Hinduism, includes actions and the intentions behind the action. The Bhagavad Gita[71] refers to the fruit of desires that give rise to the intention and the intention gives rise to actions. The positive or negative karmic outcome of the actions, intentions, and desires are binding on your soul in this life, and accumulate with the karmic outcomes of previous lives to form your next life.

This means that events in our lives are not only the result of the karmic balance we have accrued in this life, but also actions from previous lives. This explains why sometimes there is a disconnect between our actions and consequences, why bad people seem to enjoy success and prosperity, while good people suffer despite their best actions and intentions.[72]

The goal of existence is liberation from the cycle of rebirth and death and entrance into the indescribable state of moksha,[73] or liberation. While life is a temporary burden to your soul, it is the medium through which good and bad karma can be earned to help liberate your soul in the wider context of existence.

It is important to view the karmic balance, the positive and minus of negative actions and intentions accrued in this life, together with the moral and spiritual behaviour and karmic balance from previous lives. Collectively, the overall karmic balance determines how our soul will be judged and the type of rebirth we receive.

---

[66] https://www.infoplease.com/us/major-religions-world/hinduism, "Hinduism."
[67] Wikipedia, "Monotheism."
[68] "Polytheism."
[69] "Atheism."
[70] https://www.infoplease.com/us/major-religions-world/hinduism, "Hinduism."
[71] Wikipedia, "Bhagavad Gita."
[72] https://www.hinduwebsite.com/hinduism/h_karma.asp, "What Is Karma in Hinduism."
[73] Wikipedia, "Moksha."

Although Hinduism contains a broad range of philosophies, it is linked by shared concepts, and recognizable rituals. They all view karma in terms of causality[74], the result of an action is linked to the action.

The actions of a person or the intent of a person materially affect the life they lead. The actions and/or intent may be positive or negative. These are purposeful actions and deliberate actions. If the actions are unintentional or accidental, the good, or bad karma raising does not have as much weight as that arising from a deliberate or intentional act. As a result, the karmic effect may be nonexistent or have no effect on the balance of one's karma in this life or when accumulated with karma from previous lives.

For example, we often take out our car keys when we walk into a parking lot to collect our car. Sometimes, by accident, the keys will scratch the paintwork of a car we are walking past. Deliberately holding out a key, and pressing it into the paintwork to do maximum damage as we walk past, is a deliberate, intentional act and is referred to as "keying."

---

[74] "Causality."

## 10  Karma and Buddhism

**B**uddhism is founded on the teachings of a spiritual teacher, "the Buddha," "the Awakened One," the fifth to fourth century BCE.

Buddhism, as a spiritual tradition focuses on personal spiritual development and the attainment of a deep insight into the true nature of life. Buddhists seek to reach a state of nirvana, following the path of the Buddha. There are approximately 488 million followers worldwide.

In Buddhism, there is no belief in a personal god. Buddhists believe nothing is fixed or permanent and that change is always possible. The path to Enlightenment is through the practice and development of personal morality, meditation, and wisdom. Life is both endless and subject to impermanence, suffering, and uncertainty. These states are called the tilakhana[75], or the three marks of existence. Existence is endless because individuals are reincarnated repeatedly, experiencing suffering throughout many lives.

Therefore, unlike Hinduism, Buddhism practices karma as the model for our human life. In Hinduism, karma is related to rituals and prayer. In Buddhism, karma becomes the real concept that people follow and act on in their daily lives.

All Buddhist schools view karma and causality as linked. The actions of a person, or the intent of a person, materially affect the life they lead. Actions and intentions may be positive or negative. When an action is accidental, the karmic effect may be nonexistent or have no effect at all. If the action is deliberate or intentional, the karmic effect will be proportional to the action and intention and it will be good or bad. The result is referred to as the "fruit" of the action.

The karmic effect is also accumulative. At the end of life, Buddhists believe we are reincarnated into another life. The balance of the karmic value of our life, which is good karma less negative karma, is added to that of previous lives. The accumulation of karmic values and its influence on the soul's next rebirth, which is the same as Hinduism.

---

[75] "Three Marks of Existence."

A Buddhist teaching: "Do not think a minor sin will not return in your future lives."

I am the owner of my karma.
I inherit my karma.
I am born of my karma.
I am related to my karma.
I live supported by my karma.
Whatever karma I create, whether good or evil, that I shall inherit.

The Buddha, Anguttara Nikaya V.57—Upajjhatthana Sutta

## 11   Karma in Tibetan Buddhism

In all of this, Tibetan Buddhism agrees with Reincarnation and the role of Karma.

However, in Tibetan Buddhism, karma is created by physical actions, speech, and even thoughts. There is no concept of good nor bad karma—simply karma. Tibetan Buddhism teaches every creature has transmigrated helplessly since beginningless time under the influence of ignorance and that their lack of understanding has led to the performance of actions that have created connections with cyclic existence. To break this pattern, one must reorient their thinking to accord with reality. Tibetan Buddhism draws on the current human intellect for problem solving as opposed to a higher deity or power.[76]

Tibetan Buddhism believes in reincarnation and rebirth after death. The karma created in a life that has just ended is added to karma from past lives and together the accumulated karma of both affects the nature of rebirth. Karma, therefore, is continually being created within each life and across all lives our soul experiences. This is considered being a universal law of existence and has no connection to or need for abstract ideas of justice, reward, or punishment.

The Tibetan Book of the Dead contains elaborate karma purification practices and the Vajrayana[77] tradition includes how negative past karma maybe "purified" through such practices as meditation on Vajrasattva[78]. Vajrasattva is a bodhisattva in the Mahayana, Mantrayana/Vajrayana Buddhist traditions. Once the purification practices have been completed, the negative effects of karma are no longer experienced by the soul of the purified person.

In the purification process, confession of negative acts that have created negative karma is encouraged; however, renunciation of the acts is not required so long as the 4 stages of purification are completed.

1. Refuge with one hundred peaceful and wrathful deities,

2. Actual antidote with elaborate confessional acts, natural liberation practice, and Vajrasattva mantra.

3. Remorse, negative acts, genuine recollection, and resolving to never commit such negative actions again.

## 12   Karma and Bon

In Tibet, the Bon religion absorbed the ancient, verbal heritage of the Shaman. The shaman was the first human to speak with and walk with the gods. In pursuing knowledge, the shaman ascended into the heavens and descended into the underworld, where one encountered certain archetypal figures, both gods and ancestors, who initiated the individual into a death-and-rebirth transformation of one's total being, and conferred wisdom and the power to aid and protect and guide humanity, relieving its ills and suffering.[79] Bon was absorbed into Tibetan Buddhism in the

---

[76] "Karma in Tibetan Buddhism."
[77] The Mirror, "'The Tibetan Book of the Dead' and Vajrayana."
[78] Wikipedia, "Vajrasattva."
[79] http://vajranatha.com, "Ancient Tibetan Bonpo Shamanism."

eigh[th] century. Today, in 2020, approximately 12.5% of the Tibetan population is followers of Bon,[80] which is recognized by the 14th Dali Lama[81] as the sixth principal spiritual school of Tibet, along with the Nyingma, Sakya, Kagyu, Gelug and Jonang schools of Buddhism,

Bon teachings offer similar subjects, as do the other five sects of Tibetan Buddhism, with different emphases of the various deities occurring between them, or different methods of teaching. In a traditional teaching situation, the student sits at the feet of the teacher and absorbs the information as they present it in a way their culture expects, i.e., the teacher knows all. What attracts Westerners to Bon is the nature of Westerners to ask questions. Why? Why not? What about? The Bon teachings recognize this difference and respect it.[82]

Tibetan Buddhism is a form of Mahayana Buddhism stemming from the latest stages of Indian Buddhism and so is also part of the Tantric Vajrayana tradition. It thus preserves "the Tantric status quo of eighth-century India." However, it also includes native Tibetan developments and practices. In the pre-modern era, Tibetan Buddhism spread outside of Tibet primarily because of the influence of the Mongol Yuan dynasty (1271–1368), founded by Kublai Khan, which ruled China, Mongolia, and parts of Siberia. In the modern era, it has spread outside of Asia because of the efforts of the Tibetan diaspora. Apart from classical Mahayana Buddhist practices like the six perfection, Tibetan Buddhism also includes Tantric practices, such as deity yoga and the Six Dharmas of Naropa. Its primary goal is Buddhahood or rainbow body. The major language of scriptural study in this tradition is classical Tibetan.[83] [84]

Tibetans believe in karma, how a person accumulates good and bad karma in this life, and the accumulated karma of many lives through reincarnation is the same as Buddhist belief but with one exception.

## 13   Prayer Wheel—Chokhor

Chokhor is the Tibetan word for Prayer wheel, which is a common religious object in Tibet.

It is a hollow metal or wooden cylinder attached to a handle such that it can rotate freely. Attached to the cylinder is a weight on a short chain. Om Mani Padme Hung mantras are printed or etched in relief on the cylinder. By manipulating the handle and cylinder, the weight can spin the cylinder.

It is believed that one rotation of the cylinder bearing the mantra is the equivalent of saying the mantra at one time. This practice helps the user accumulate merit—good karma, which replaces any negative karma they have accumulated.

Religious exercise is part of Tibetan life. People turn the wheel day and night while walking or resting whenever their right hands are free while murmuring the same mantra. Buddhists turn the wheel clockwise. Bon followers turn the wheel counterclockwise.

---

[80] Wikipedia, "Religion in Tibet."
[81] Ligmincha International, "Message from Dalai Lama.Pdf."
[82] 60208 https://www.taosnews.com/stories/ancient-wisdom-of-the-himalayas, "Ancient Wisdom of the Himalayas."
[83] Wikipedia, "Tibetan Buddhism."
[84] "Karma in Tibetan Buddhism."

One common image from Tibet is large prayer wheels arranged in a line along a wall outside a shrine or Buddhist temple with people walking along the line and spinning the drums with their right hand. The same mantras are etched or stamped into the surface of the payer wheel, producing the same beneficial merit for the person spinning the wheels. Even larger prayer wheels powered by water, fire, or wind produce the same effect, but powering the wheel with one of the five elements of water and wind produced positive karma to all who touch them.

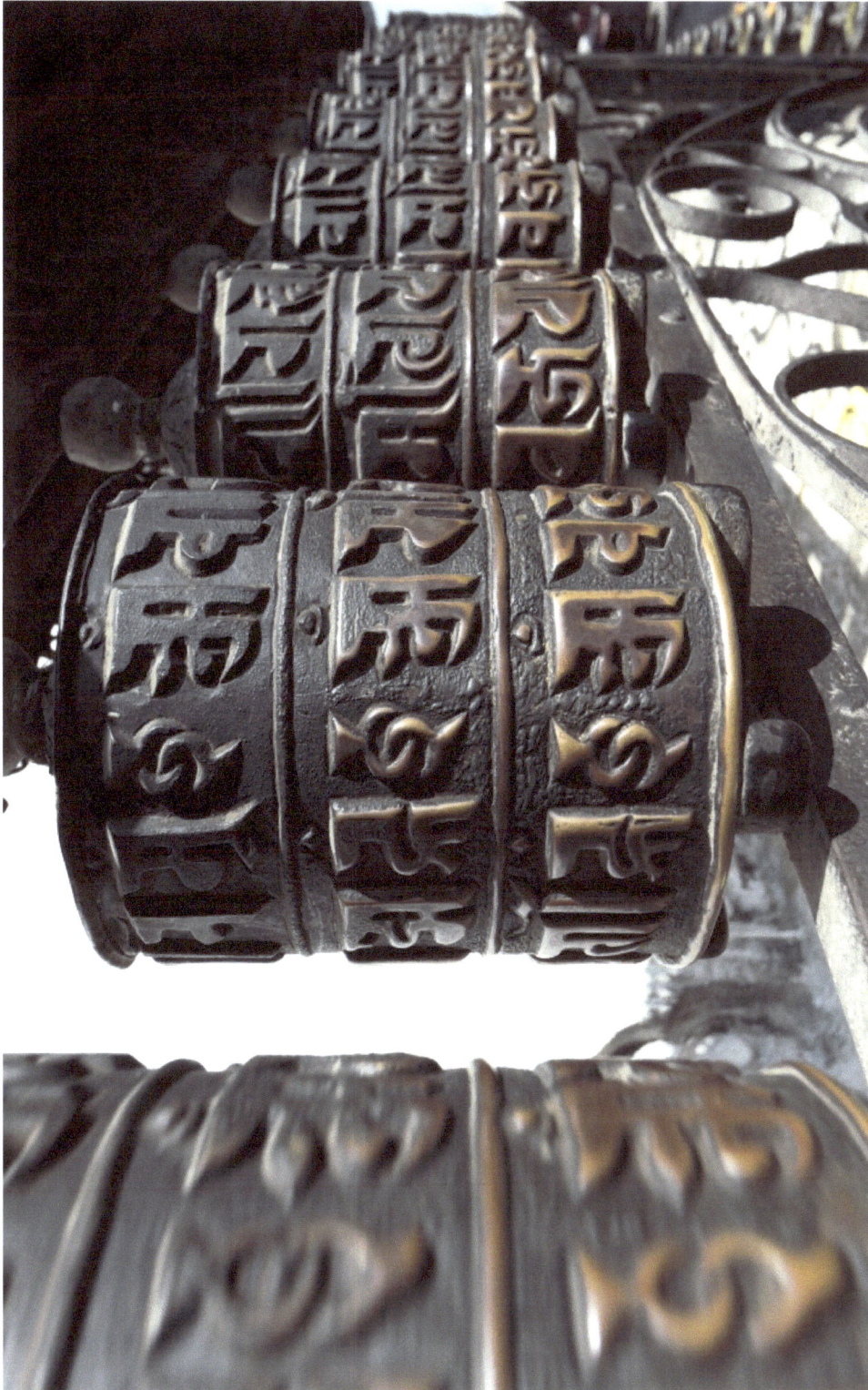

*Figure 2. Large Prayer Wheels at a Monastery*

## 14   Karma and Jainism

A ll Hindu, Jain and Buddhist schools view karma and casualties, or the result of an action as linked. The actions of a person, or the intent of a person, materially affect karma or the merit they accumulate through life as well as influencing the type of life they lead.

Jains believe in the philosophy of karma, reincarnation of the worldly soul, hell, and heaven as a punishment or reward for one's deeds, and liberation Nirvana or Moksha of the self from life's misery of birth and death in a way similar to Hindu and Buddhist beliefs. Though there are multiple similarities in these religions, there are some major portions of the belief system that remain unique to each religion. For instance, the Jain philosophy believes that the universe and all its entities, such as souls and physical matter, are eternal. They have no beginning or end, no one has created them and no one can destroy them.[85]

Jains do not believe that there is a supernatural power or God who does favour us if we please him. Jains rely a great deal on self-effort and self-initiative, for both—their worldly requirements and their redemption. Jainism appeals to common sense. Jains accept only those things that can be explained and reasoned. Jains believe that each living being is a master of his/her own destiny. [86]

---

[85] jainbelief.com, "Jainism."
[86] Ibid.

## 15 Karma and Sikhism

God is the creator of the first Karma, the origin of the universe, and the ultimate destroyer of Karma.

Our present life results from past Karma; our present Karma determines our future life. Karma operates in this life and successive ones. The law of Karma does not cease to operate after death, because death is just a matter of physical disintegration, and has no effect on the soul, which survives.[87]

Good or evil, by frequent repetition, leaves their impression on a person's character. A man doing wicked deeds continuously will turn into an evil character. This produces various states of mind, like anxiety, fear and guilt, all of which will cause pain and suffering for the individual in this life. [88]

Although Karma may influence the reincarnation of a soul, nothing is preordained. A person keeps their free will and a person's actions will determine who he is in their current life. God, as the Ruler of the Universe, controls the over-all destiny of an individual. Like the prodigal son, sinners turn to him only as the last resort. [89]

Sikhism made two modifications to the theory of Karma.

- Efforts by the individual are necessary for improving his own condition. Man handles his lot. He must not blame God for his destiny. He must think of the present and the future.

- Second, Karma can be changed by prayer and the Grace of God.

---

[87] https://www.allaboutsikhs.com/sikhism-faqs/sikhism-faqswhat-is-karma, "Sikhism Faqs What Is Karma?."
[88] Ibid.
[89] Ibid.

## 16   Karma and Taoism

Taoist Karma does not follow Buddhist or Hindu beliefs.

Taoism was built on earlier shamanic and proto religious divination practices, which likely originated outside of China and were carried by various ancient migrations. All Taoists believe the movement of the cosmos determines the affairs of the earth and that in order to change your destiny, you must align correctly with the terrestrial and cosmic changing of yin and yang.

In the notion of Karma, there is the concept of good and bad karma, and by implication, there is justice, some way to determine what good and bad karma and how to weigh one against another. This leads to the desire for a universe that provides divine law that mandates these things. Karma for Buddhism and Hinduism expresses that desire.

Tao is all things and to all people it is the same. It is in everything we experience good or evil, creation or destruction, birth or death, beauty or ugliness.

Tao does not favour or give more weight to something or determines one thing is good and another bad. Humans have free will and must use it to create a desirable world. The Tao will not do it for us because that would violate our free will.

To Taoist karma, you must understand and agree the universe is driven by your choices and our free will.

## 17   Karma and Orthodox Christianity

**D**o not be deceived. God is not mocked: for whatever a man sows that he will also reap. Galatians 6.7

- They sow the wind and reap the whirlwind. Hosea 8.7

Orthodox Christianity does to accept reincarnation. "It is appointed to men to die once, but then the judgment" Hebrews 9.27.

As a result, a Christian follower believes they have one life, die once, and will then receive judgment for their actions in that life. If judgment is to suffer pain and penalties because of their actions, it is carried out in the same body as they were committed in. There is no escape. We live with ourselves; passions defect to eternity.

Through the theory of salvation, embracing and adhering to the Truth and Life of Jesus Christ is the only way to escape the consequences of our evil deeds.

## 18   Karma and Catholicism

The Roman Catholic Church does not believe in Karma.

The Catholic Church, sometimes referred to as the Roman Catholic Church, is the largest Christian church, with approximately 1.3 billion baptized Catholics worldwide as of 2018. As the world's oldest and largest continuously functioning international institutions, it has played a prominent role in the history and development of Western civilization.[90]

The Catholic Church shared communion with the Eastern Orthodox Church, hence the separate section on the Orthodox church, until the East—West Schism in 1054, which disputed the authority of the pope. Earlier splits within the church occurred after the Council of Ephesus 431 and the Council of Chalcedon 451. However, a few Eastern Churches remained in communion with Rome, and portions of some others established communion in the 15th century and later, forming what are called the Eastern Catholic Churches.[91] In the 16th century, the Reformation led to Protestantism.[92]

Depending on who is in a discussion on the concept of Karma, the belief may be pagan, and anyone who believes in it believes in false idols. However, the same person may say that Karma itself is not evil and that a person who carries out good work, engages in good behaviour and expresses good intentions will create good for themselves.

In Christian Philosophical Theology, there are two views of religion. The eastern view that includes and is founded on karma and reincarnation and the western one is based on Abrahamic philosophy, which speaks to a religion of grace and salvation.

A karmic approach says that, by a cosmic spiritual law, we are punished or rewarded according to our moral activities. If we do bad things, we will suffer, either in this life or a life to come. And if we do good things, we will be rewarded, again either here or in there. Karma might not be immediate, as is the law of gravity but in the long run, people are rewarded or punished according to merit. And this satisfies our sense of fairness and justice.[93]

Removing the belief in reincarnation, all our efforts, and the judgment of what we do, and what we deserve as a result are concentrated on this single life. One life and then judgment.

A religion of grace teaches that *all* people are sinners and hence deserving of punishment, but that God, out of sheer generosity, gives them what they don't deserve. Think of one of the most popular lines in Christian poetry: "Amazing grace, how sweet the sound that saved a wretch like me." In terms of a karmic religion, wretches deserve a wretched fate, and it would be unfair for wicked people to be given a substantial gift. But devotees of a religion of grace exult in this generosity. [94]

Simply put, the Roman Catholic Church does not believe in Karma. Salvation through belief and worship of Jesus Christ has more value than Karma by itself.

---

[90] Wikipedia, "Catholic Church."
[91] Ibid.
[92] Ibid.
[93] https://www.ncregister.com/blog/robert-barron/grace-or-karma, "Grace or Karma."
[94] Ibid.

## 19  Karma and Islam

**M**uslims are people who follow or practise Islam, a monotheistic Abrahamic religion. Muslims consider the Quran, their holy book, to be the verbatim word of God as revealed to the Islamic prophet and messenger Muhammad. Most Muslims also follow the teachings and practices of Muhammad (Sunnah) as recorded in traditional accounts hadith. "Muslim" is an Arabic word meaning "submitter" to God.[95]

The beliefs of Muslims include that God Allah is eternal, transcendent and absolutely one tawhid[96]; that God is incomparable and self-sustaining, and neither begets nor was begotten; that Islam is the complete and universal version of a primordial faith that has been revealed before through many prophets, including Abraham, Ishmael, Isaac, Moses, and Jesus; that these previous messages and revelations have been partially changed or corrupted over time tahrif[97] and that the Quran is the final unaltered revelation from God's Final Testament. [98]

The religious practices of Muslims are enumerated in the Five Pillars of Islam: [99]

- The declaration of faith shahadah,

- daily prayers salat,

- fasting during the month of Ramadan sawm,

- almsgiving zakat,

- pilgrimage to Mecca hajj at least once in a lifetime.

Karma doesn't exist in Islam; instead, there is Kifarah. What you give you will get back. If you are good, good will come to you. If you are bad, bad things will come to you. If someone wrongs you, be patient, Allah is fair; he has a plan for them.

Obviously, this is very similar to Karma, except that Allah, or God, will address the wrong.

---

[95] Wikipedia, "Muslims."
[96] "Tawhid."
[97] "Tahrif."
[98] "Muslims."
[99] Ibid.

## 20  Karma and Protestantism

**P**rotestantism is the second-largest form of Christianity with 800 million to 1 billion adherents worldwide, or about 37% of all Christians. It originated with the 16th-century Reformation, a movement against what its followers perceived to be errors in the Catholic Church. Protestants reject the Roman Catholic doctrine of papal supremacy and sacraments, but disagree among themselves regarding the actual presence of Christ in the Eucharist. They emphasize the priesthood of all believers, justification by faith alone, sola fide, rather than also by good works, and the highest authority of the Bible alone rather than also with sacred tradition in faith and morals (sola scriptura). The "five solae" summarize basic theological differences in opposition to the Roman Catholic Church.[100]

The political separation of the Church of England from the pope under King Henry VIII began Anglicanism, bringing England and Wales into this broad Reformation movement.[101]

Although the concepts of resentment and karma play important parts in society, Buddhism, Jainism, Sikhism, and Taoism, etc., hold those as key concepts, whereas they are nonexistent in Protestantism, as they refer to those concepts as sin.

Protestantism is therefore a religion of Salvation, as are The Roman Catholic and Orthodox Christian religions.

---

[100] Wikipedia, "Protestantism."
[101] Ibid.

## 22   Karma in the West

In the west, karma is often understood by the simple expression, "what goes around, comes around?" as said by a friend of mine looking at the deliberate keying of a door in her Mercedes. The bad karma—physical action and spiritual intent of the individual who carried out this malicious act will return to them in some unspecified and unknown way. It is not important that she is aware of when or how karma addresses the malicious action.

Another slightly different phasing of the belief in karma was another friend who, when asked about their response to a negative action directed at them, said simply, "I'll let karma take care of it." Karmic actions and responses can be thought of as a seedling that will inevitably grow and ripen, and the resulting fruit will either be tasty and delicious or it will be bitter and tasteless.

In both cases, I would say most cases where karma is left to address wrongdoing, the recipient of bad karma will not be involved in any personal retribution aimed at the wrongdoer.

While both examples deal with malicious acts, karma can also be said of good deeds. A person delivering a good deed to a person will receive good fortune in their lives. But again, the form and timing of good karma will go unknown by the person who received it.

The effect of a good or bad deed may be material, moral, or emotional—that is, it affects one's happiness and unhappiness. The effect of karma need not be immediate; the effect of karma can be later in one's current life, and in some schools, it extends to future lives.[102]

In all these examples, the person receiving good or bad karma would be a Christian who does not accept the existence of karma or karmic actions and reciprocity.

In Science, we see karma in Newton's Third Law of Motion, according to which every action has an equal and opposite reaction is "proof" that it exists.

---

[102] https://en.wikipedia.org/wiki/Karma, "Karma."

## 23 Karma in New Age

**A**n eclectic group of cultural attitudes arising in late 20th century Western society that is adapted from those of a variety of ancient and modern cultures that emphasize beliefs such as reincarnation, holism, pantheism, and occultism outside the mainstream, and that advance alternative approaches to spirituality, right living, and health.[103]

New Age encompasses a very broad range of spiritual or religious beliefs which developed in the Western World during the 1970s. The New Age philosophy is non-unified and includes beliefs and practices from eastern and western religious traditions, as well as a holistic approach to health, motivational and positive psychology research. New Age is so broad because the general development of human understanding started to coalesce across an amazingly wide variety of human experience and empowered people to castoff organized religious structures and organizations. New agers, as they are called, don't limit their belief system to one particular doctrine.

Typically, the belief systems seen under the term New Age adopt a holistic form of divinity that includes, but is not limited to, the universe, including human beings, and contains a strong emphasis on the spiritual authority of the individual's self. This is accompanied by a common belief in a wide variety of semi-divine non-human entities, such as angels and masters, with whom humans can communicate, particularly through the form of channelling.

Although analytically often considered being religious, those involved typically prefer the designation of spiritual or Mind, Body and Spirit and rarely use the term New Age themselves. Many scholars of the subject refer to it as the New Age movement, although others contest this term and suggest that it is better seen as a milieu or zeitgeist.

New Age has antecedents that stretch back to southern Europe in Late Antiquity—between the 3rd and eighth centuries AD. Following the Age of Enlightenment in 18th century Europe, new esoteric ideas developed in response to the development of scientific rationality. Scholars call this new esoteric trend occultism, and this occultism was a key factor in the worldview's development from which the New Age emerged.

New Age literature often refers to benevolent non-human spirits with whom humans can communicate, particularly through the form of channelling. The belief system contains a strong focus on healing using forms of alternative medicine, which includes a strong connection to semi-divine non-human entities. New Age contains the notion that spirituality and science can be unified. As a result, New Age places Meditation alongside Quantum Physics.

New Age spirituality or New Age religion is often used instead of simply New age. New Age followers usually view references to spirituality and religion negatively, seeing the terms as "coded" defences to monolithic organized religions, such as Christianity in particular. Some New Age adherents self-identify as a New Age member of an established religious group, i.e., Christianity, Judaism, or Buddhism, where some of the religious doctrine is accepted and other parts are not.

---

[103] Merriam-Webster, "Definition of New Age."

For example, Christianity does not accept reincarnation or karma because true Christians adhere to the message of salvation in Jesus Christ and the Bible. However, a New Age Christian believer might discard this and accept reincarnation and karma in their hybrid New Age/Christian view.

With New Age flexibility and having no central doctrine, no central authority, and able to ingest all religious traditions, or parts of those traditions to create a new whole, reincarnation, and karma are both accepted and both "operate as described" in previous sections.

## 24   Karma in Science

**P**erhaps the simplest illustration of Karma is Sir Isaac Newton's[104] Third Law of Motion[105].

- For every action, there is an equal and opposite reaction.

In terms of karma, this would mean that a good deed by someone would be returned to them at the same value. Of course, a wrongdoer would receive an equal and opposite wrong. A more scientific expression of "what goes around, comes around."

C. C. Jung,[106] in his view of World Religions,[107] was quite agnostic regarding karma, though he was careful to distinguish between metempsychosis and reincarnation, since the former did not imply continuity of personality while the latter did.

Jung's fiercest criticisms of Indian religions were reserved for their facile dismissal of evil as an illusion. Using meditation or yoga as a method of escape engendered scathing comments about maharishi and gurus, who attained "serenity" by ignoring the material world. [108]

The Jungian system takes precedence over the religions of the world and they are judged by the extent to which they conform to and facilitate the Jungian drive to psychic wholeness.

The extreme emphasis on symbols within Jungian thought enables religious symbols to be redefined, reinterpreted and, where necessary, reinvented from events originally seen as literally. Although Jung is pro-religion in the sense that, unlike Freud, he treats it as a vehicle for meaning and evidence of the more than merely sexual nature of human beings; he is religious on his own terms. Although Freud considers religion to be almost entirely a neurosis and an illusion, Jung sees it as evidence of realities about human beings and the world, which its doctrines and dogmas only indirectly address. A serious Jungian approach to world religions would be at odds with a strictly phenomenological approach, for example, since Jung quickly goes beyond the consciousness of the believer into his own hermeneutic, while phenomenology, particularly of a strictly Husserlian sort, stays as close as it can within the parameters of the believer's perceptions. [109]

---

[104] Wikipedia, "Isaac Newton."
[105] https://www.physicsclassroom.com/class/newtlaws/Lesson-4/Newton-s-Third-Law, "Newton's Third Law of Motion."
[106] Wikipedia, "Carl Jung."
[107] https://glyndwr.repository.guildhe.ac.uk/246/1/fulltext.pdf, "Jung and World Religions."
[108] Ibid.
[109] Ibid.

## 25   Karma Fruit Bearing or the Result

We have mentioned this in previous sections, but for clarity; we are going into the concept of Karma fruit bearing to separate it from a religion.

The consequence or effects of one's karma can be described in two forms: phala[110] and samskara[111]. A phala, literally, fruit or result is the visible or invisible effect that is typically immediate or within the current life. In contrast, samskara[112] is invisible effects, produced by the actor because of karma, transforming the agent and affecting his or her ability to be happy or unhappy in this life and future ones. The theory of karma is often presented in samskara[113].

Fruit-bearing Karma is Karma that has immediate consequences during our lifetime. By constantly berating and criticizing people around us, we find that we have no close friends and are extremely lonely with no one to turn to in a time of need. This is a consequence we have brought on ourselves. It is immediate.

Karma is not only the bad; however, it is the sum of everything we bring into our lives and that we empty into this world. Berating and criticizing people around us may result from our upbringing and experiences, but it can also be a consequence of past lives. Karma means that the person who is unable to conceive in this lifetime, but is caring and loving, will find themselves with all the families they could want in the next.

Karma is personal to each of us. It cannot be wished on anyone else, no matter how dearly we would like karma to be visited on someone. The fact is that if we could wish or transfer karma to another person, the act would be bad karma for us. We would have to pay karmically, emotionally, and spiritually for doing so. We would have a reckoning with this action and deed.

Ultimately, everyone must face the consequences of the things they have done in their life, even if it is only at their death. We never truly know what is going on in a person's life unless we are walking in their shoes. Think of the number of celebrities who "had it all" that committed suicide.

---

[110] Wikipedia, "Phala."
[111] "Samskara."
[112] Ibid.
[113] Ibid.

## 26   Karmic Accumulation and Debt

**K**arma of the spirit has a significant role to play in reincarnation. Our soul accumulates karma in different lives; the resulting karmic balance of our soul through different lives affects nature and type of our rebirth. Accumulated Karma is the Karma that transfers from lifetime to lifetime.

Karma is a two-way street. If I punch you in the arm and hurt you, but it is accidental, the effect on my karma will be less than if I had punched you intending to hurt you. Your karma is affected because you trusted me and did not expect or accept that receiving a punch in the arm is acceptable. The break in your trust that I will not punch you in the arm is your karma. The intention to hurt you and the action is mine.

We have all encountered people at work, sometimes supervisors or managers, who represented ideas like theirs in meetings or two higher levels of management. Their karma is that they do not to the work and knowingly misrepresent what it is they have taken from someone else.

Sometimes this is a symbiotic[114] relationship. I do the work, and knowingly allow you to represent it as yours but I receive benefit or karma, such as a better workstation, chair, computer or I may leave early.

In my experience, the misrepresentation, and the bad karma of it are usually secretive and discovered accidentally.

More serious is the loss of your personal power. Someone has taken away from you something that is important for your wellbeing.

Some things can be material, such as the theft or vandalizing a vehicle. My friend, who had the door on her Mercedes keyed, felt the loss in her karma for the long hours of work and travel away from her family that had allowed her to "have something nice." The damage was repaired, but the cost was not just financial, it was more hours of effort and travel and a delay in renovating a room in her home she had planned because of the cost of repairing the car. She also felt the hurt over her loss of control over being unable to prevent the damage.

Expressing who we are through our karma is material for removing or paying back a past life karmic debt. The act of depriving another of their life, intentional murder or by allowing someone to die through lack of action is depriving another soul of its ability to express its karma in this world and accumulate good and bad karma for its rebirth.

Saving a life, and the good karma arising from the act, adds to your karma in this life and repays a past karmic debt where your soul has been involved in the death of another.

This raises the question of our connection with other souls. As we are reincarnated, we take on a different physical appearance. Acts such as taking or giving life can represent a connection between the souls in each person from past lives.

---

114 https://www.merriam-webster.com/dictionary/symbiotic, "Definition of Symbiotic."

We are all interconnected and how we choose to exercise our karma and affect the interconnection for good or bad. Lying so that another is found guilty and incarcerated unfairly. Or denying a person or group of people their freedom and ability to enhance, experience, and enrich their souls. Is bad karma on a much bigger, grander scale with no personal connection to those affected by our karma?

The counter-argument to these acts of karma is that the person or group who is being denied freedom and the ability to enrich their souls experience it. That the members of the group denied their freedom should struggle, perhaps fruitlessly, and endure through confinement and the inability to enrich their soul and karma.

Causing injury to another, giving them a power tool such as a chain saw to cut wood without correct instruction or knowing that the safety mechanism does not work properly and they seriously injury themselves, perhaps a bad scar, or loss of a limb affects the person and their soul for the rest of this physical life. But it also affects how others see that person as well as how the person who was injured can represent themselves. If you give a neighbour a ladder to clean their eves trough, knowing it is unsafe, and they fall, and have a serious injury, leaving them in a wheelchair for the rest of their lives, your karma must deal with your neighbour's inability to live their life fully as well as the distortion the wheelchair places on their lives—it is unfortunate that society focuses on disability rather than what the disabled person offers.

## 27   What is the Soul?

### 27.1   Etymology

In Modern English, the word "soul" is derived from Old English sáwol, sáwel, was first attested in the 8th century poem Beowulf v. 2820 and in the Vespasian Psalter 77.50. It is cognate with other German and Baltic terms for the same idea, including Gothic saiwala, Old High German sêula, sêla, Old Saxon sêola, Old Low Franconian sêla, sîla, Old Norse sála, and Lithuanian siela. Deeper etymology of the Germanic word is unclear.[115]

The original concept behind the Germanic root is thought to mean, "coming from or belonging to the sea (or lake)", because of the Germanic and pre-Celtic belief in souls emerging from and returning to sacred lakes, Old Saxon sêola (soul) compared to Old Saxon sêo (sea). [116]

### 27.2   A Definition

The word "soul" can refer to the Spirit of God. Or, if the person speaking to me does not want to refer to "God," just "Spirit." It exists in each individual; it is an ever-existing, ever-conscious, ever-new bliss.

Identifying the Soul with the physical body and becomes the nature of the individual. References to "spiritual progress" or "soul evolution" use this definition, because the soul that is aware of its true identity as part of God is already perfect. Souls only develop or progress in the sense that they go from identifying with their physical bodies to identifying with God. This can also be called the ego.

### 27.3   Dictionary Definition

Merriam-Webster Dictionary[117]

- the immaterial essence, animating principle, or actuating cause of an individual life

- the spiritual principle embodied in human beings, all rational and spiritual beings, or the universe

- Capitalized, Christian Science: GOD senses

- a person's total self

- an active or essential part

- of a moving spirit: LEADER

- the moral and emotional nature of human beings

---

[115] Wikipedia, "Soul."

[116] Ibid.

[117] Merriam-Webster Dictionary, "Definition of Soul by Merriam-Webster."

- the quality that arouses emotion and sentiment

- spiritual or moral force: FERVOUR

## 27.4 Atman—Hinduism

Atman is a Sanskrit word that means inner self, spirit, or soul. In Hindu philosophy, especially in the Vedanta school of Hinduism, Atman is the first principle: the true self of an individual beyond identification with phenomena, the essence of an individual. In order to attain liberation (moksha), a human being must gain self-knowledge, which is to realize that one's true self is identical to the transcendent self-Brahman.

The six orthodox schools of Hinduism believe that there is Atman (soul, self) in every being. This is a major point of difference with the Buddhist doctrine of Anatta, which holds that there is no unchanging soul or self.

## 27.5 Theological Soul

Soul and the spirit are the two primary immaterial parts that Scripture ascribes to humanity.[118] The word spirit refers only to the immaterial facet of humanity. Human beings have a spirit, but we are not spirits. However, the soul and spirit are often used interchangeably; the primary distinction between soul and spirit is that in men and women the soul has animated life, or is the seat of the senses, desires, affections, and appetites.

The soul, in many religious, philosophical, and mythological traditions, is the ethereal essence of a living being. The soul or psyche comprises the mental abilities of a living being: reason, character, feeling, consciousness, memory, perception, thinking, etc. Depending on the philosophical system, a soul can either be mortal or immortal.[119] The soul is alive, physically and eternally. The spirit can be alive, as with believers (1 Peter 3:18), or dead as unbelievers are (Colossians 2:13; Ephesians 2:4-5).

Believers in Jesus Christ and his role in salvation respond to the things that come from the Spirit of God, understanding and discerning them spiritually. The spirit allows us to connect, or not, with God. Our spirits relate to His Spirit, either accepting his promptings and conviction, proving that we belong to him (Romans 8:16) or resisting him and proving that we do not have a spiritual life (Acts 7:51).

The spirit is the element in humanity that gives us the ability to have an intimate relationship with God. Whenever the word spirit is used, it refers to the immaterial part of humanity that "connects" with God, who himself is spirit (John 4:24).

Judaism and Christianity teach that only human beings have immortal souls, although immortality is disputed within Judaism and the concept of immortality may have been influenced by Plato.

The "origin of the soul" has provided a vexing question in Christianity. The major theories put forward include soul creationism, traducianism, and pre-existence. According to soul creationism,

---

[118] GotQuestions.org, "What Is the Difference between the Soul and Spirit of Man?."
[119] Wikipedia, "Soul."

God creates each individual soul created directly, either at the moment of conception or some later time. According to traducianism, the soul comes from the parents by natural generation. According to the pre-existence theory, the soul exists before the moment of conception. There have been differing thoughts regarding whether human embryos have souls from conception, or whether there is a point between conception and birth where the fetus gains a soul, consciousness, and/or personhood. Stances in this question might play a role in judgments on the morality of abortion.[120]

The most basic meaning of "soul" is "life," there is no distinction whether it refers to physical or eternal life. Jesus asks what it profits a man to gain the entire world and lose his soul, referring to his eternal life (Matthew 16:26). Both Old and New Testaments reiterate we are to love God completely, with the whole "soul," which refers to everything that is in us that makes us alive (Deuteronomy 6:4-5; Mark 12:30). Whenever the word "soul" is used, it can refer to the whole person, whether physically alive or in the afterlife.

The soul is our source of absolute uniqueness, a place within that connects you not only to your own value and essence, but to the value and essence of every other living being. This is limiting; we will get back to that later.

---

[120] Ibid.

## 27.6  Where Is the Soul in the Physical Body?

Debate on "where" the soul is in a physical body is a large and disruptive discussion topic. Mostly because we do not have a suitable definition by which to recognize the soul if we are lucky enough or astute enough to find it!

- Descartes: The pineal gland is a tiny organ in the centre of the brain that played an important role in Descartes's philosophy. He regarded it as the principal seat of the soul and the place in which all our thoughts are formed.[121]

- Leonardo da Vinci used his experience in anatomy to hypothesize that the soul was in the optic chiasm, near the third ventricle of the brain. His views were supported by observations of change in perception following disturbances to that area of the brain.[122]

- Aristotle in De Anima (On the Soul) suggests that the organs of the body are required for the soul to interact with. Unlike Plato, Aristotle believed the soul's existence was not separate from the human body; thus the soul could not be immortal. Similarly, to Plato, however, Aristotle believed the soul is composed of three parts: the vegetative, sensitive, and rational. Growth and reproduction result from the vegetative soul, and are found in all organisms. The sensitive soul, however, allows for sensation and movement in humans and animals. Third, the rational is exclusive to humans, and allows for rational thought.[123]

## 27.7  Ensoulment

After considering "where" the soul can be found in the body, how does it get there, when does it arrive?

In religion, ensoulment is the moment at which a human being gains a soul.[124] [125] Some religions say that a soul is newly created within a developing child and others, especially in religions that believe in reincarnation[126], that the soul is pre-existing and added at a particular stage of development.
In the time of Aristotle, it was widely believed that the human soul entered the forming body at 40 days (male embryos) or 90 days (female embryos), and quickening showed a soul. Other religious views are that ensoulment happens at the moment of conception; or when the child takes the first breath after being born; at the formation of the nervous system and brain; at the first brain activity (e.g., heartbeat); or when the fetus can survive independently of the uterus (viability).[127]

The concept is closely related to debates on the morality of abortion and the morality of contraception. Religious belief that human life has an innate sacredness have motivated many

---

[121] Stanford Encyclopedia of Philosophy, "Descartes and the Pineal Gland."
[122] Wikipeda, "History of the Location of the Soul."
[123] Ibid.
[124] Wikipedia, "Ascended Master."
[125] https://en.wikipedia.org/wiki/The_City_of_God, "The City of God."
[126] http://healerofheartsandminds.com, "Reincarnation, Past Lives, Suffering and the Bible, a Shaman's Views."
[127] Wikipedia, "Ascended Master."

statements by spiritual leaders of various traditions over the years. However, the three matters are not exactly parallel, given that various figures have argued that some kind of life without a soul, in various contexts, still has a moral worth that must be considered. [128]

## 27.8  Shamanic Soul

The Catholic theologian Thomas Aquinas[129] attributed "soul" to all organisms but argued that only human souls are immortal. Other religions, most notably Hinduism and Jainism, hold that all living things, from the smallest bacterium, to the largest mammals, are the souls themselves and have their physical representative, the body, in the world. The actual self is the soul; the body is simply a mechanism to experience the karma of that life. Thus, if we see a tiger, then there is a self-conscious identity or soul living in it, and a physical representative of the whole body of the tiger, which is observable in the world. Some teach that even non-biological entities such as rivers and mountains possess souls. This belief is called animism.[130]

Animism is a major part of the shamanic worldview and an understanding of what this world represents. Shamans often work by being able to reach a different level of consciousness or awareness that allows them to speak to the spirits of the natural world, who can then provide them with knowledge and information. Shamanism often relies pretty heavily on animistic ideas with most shamanistic practices, but not all but animism can exist without shamanism.

The soul is the principle of life, feeling, thought, and action in humans. In some religions, it is believed that when the person dies, although their body is no longer alive, their spirit or soul moves on to another world. The soul in religion is needed for reincarnation, which is clear in Hinduism and Buddhism, where, when we die, our souls come back to take over the body of any living matter. Souls are not only clear in religion, but in philosophy.

---

[128] Ibid.
[129] Wikipedia, "Robert Thurman."
[130] "Soul."

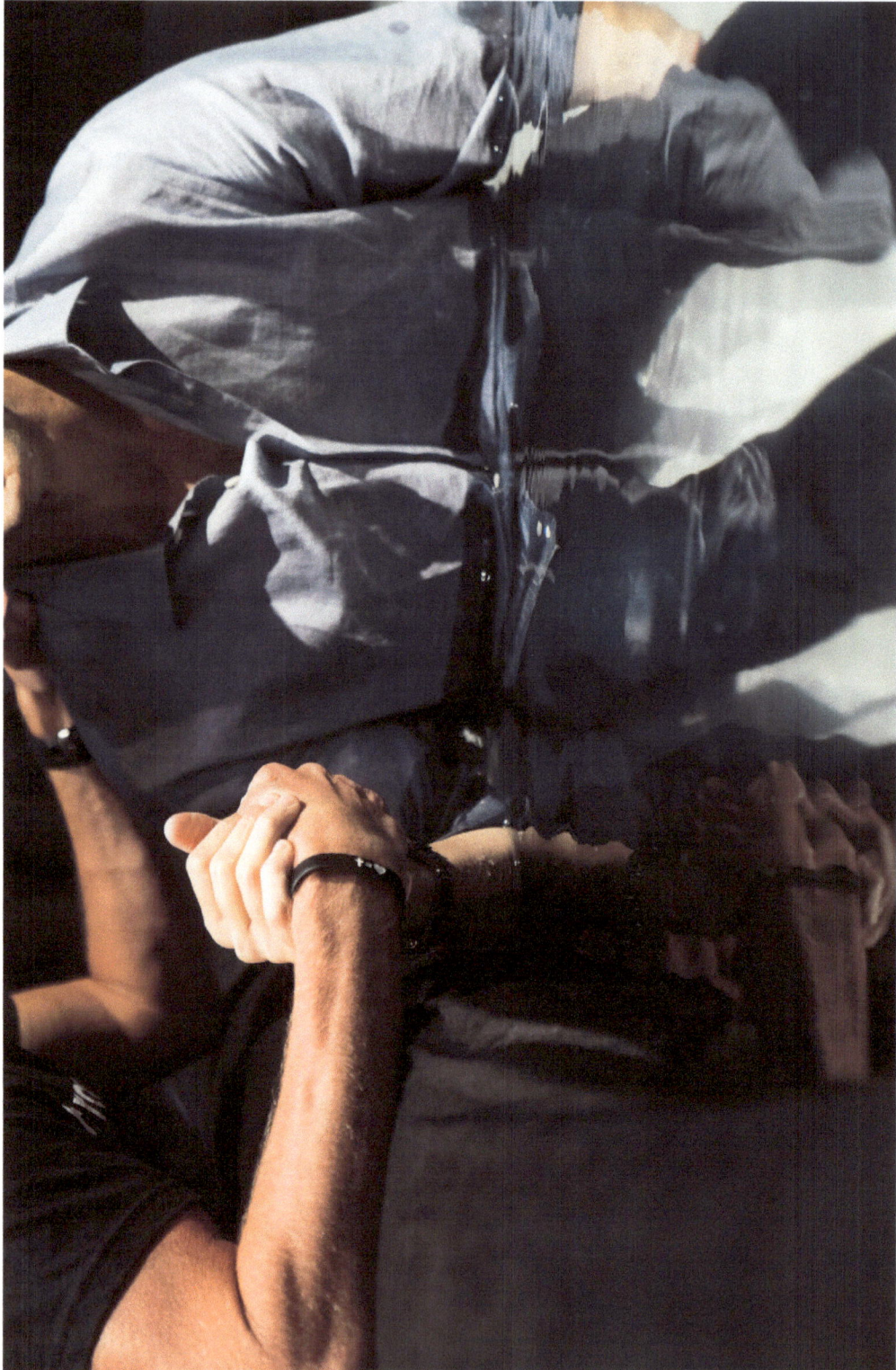

Figure 3. Rebirth. Photo by kaleb tapp on Unsplash

## 28  Rebirth

In some schools of Buddhism, Bardo, antarabhava, or chuu is an intermediate or liminal state between death and rebirth—reincarnation. Reincarnation into another life, as a different being, is the philosophical or religious concept that the non-physical essence of a living being starts a new life in a different physical form or body after biological death. It is also called rebirth or transmigration.[131]

The Buddhist view is that a person's actions shape his or her own future existence and ultimately determine into which of the six realms they will take rebirth following death. This means that people who do not believe in God but do-good deeds during their lives will not go to hell. The Buddhist theory of karma holds that you are what you do. Even those who don't believe in the Buddha will reap the rewards in a future life if they do well and avoid all harmful acts. Buddhist karma tells us that positive action results in beneficial reaction, whereas negative action results in unwanted reaction. Therefore, it is often said that karma follows a person like a shadow.[132]

It is important to remember that when the soul consciousness leaves the physical body, it may remain for a while around the body, in a favourite room, or around a favourite person without connecting to the dead body. When the soul leaves its body, it will see it and not connect with the meaning of it. This sets it apart from the Out of Body Experiences, where there is a connection, a necessary connection to what is still a physically living body.

The connection of soul disappeared in the dissolution stage of dying. However, death is usually a very emotional environment. People are crying, expressing themselves emotionally, naming the body, recalling his life and his qualities, his virtues, etc. Maybe competitors or people who did not like him are criticizing, complaining, and glad that he is no longer physically around. But all of this, the good and the bad, are gone. Dissolution has restarted the counter: the memories of consciousness. A Shaman will be called if the emotions of those who knew the soul in physical form are so strong, they hold the soul to the physical realm, causing reconnection with them. Later, if the soul disconnects but does not complete the process of rebirth, it may wander the physical realm, connecting to people with which it has no purpose, but sometimes injury those living souls and consciousness.

### 28.1  Is Rebirth Simultaneous?

A controversial subject I rebirth is whether it is simultaneous with death. According to Abhidhamma[133], rebirth or conception, as it is known, takes place immediately after the death of a being with no intermediate state. Some others believe that a person, after his death, would develop into a spirit form for a certain number of days before rebirth takes place. Another interpretation regarding the same belief is that it is not the spirit, but the deceased person's consciousness or mental energy remaining in space, supported by his own mental energies of craving and attachment. However, eventually rebirth must take place. The spirit petas, who are beings born in spirit form, are unfortunately living beings and their lives in the spirit form are not permanent. It is also rebirth which is temporary.[134]

---

131 https://en.wikipedia.org/wiki/The_City_of_God, "The City of God."
132 https://link.springer.com/article/10.1186/s40613-015-0016-2, "On the Naturalization of Karma and Rebirth."
133 Wikipedia, "Bhagavad Gita."
134 https://www.budsas.org/ebud/whatbudbeliev/96.htm, "What Buddhists Believe - Rebirth."

A concept many people have difficulty with is that, in the process of rebirth, a human being may be reborn as an animal and an animal may be reborn as a human being. The animal nature of the mind and the animal way of life adopted by him can cause him to be reborn as an animal. The condition and behaviour of the mind handle the next existence. A person who is born in animal form, owing to certain mental abuses during a previous birth, could be reborn as a human being if that animal has committed none serious evil acts. Some animals are very intelligent and understanding. This is clear evidence to prove that they are tending towards a human life. A person who is reborn as an animal can again be born as a human being when the bad karma which conditioned his birth as an animal is spent and the good karma which was stored. [135]

It is foolish to waste human existence along with the conducive conditions that we enjoy in free societies and the opportunity that we have to practise the Dharma[136]. It is extremely important that having this opportunity we make use of it. If we cannot practise the Dharma in this life, there is no way of knowing where in the six realms we will be reborn, and when we shall have such a chance again. We must strive to free ourselves from the cycle of rebirth because failing to do so means that we will continue to circle endlessly among these six realms of existence. When the karma, wholesome or unwholesome, that causes us to be born in any of the six realms is exhausted, rebirth will occur, and we will find ourselves again in another realm. In fact, it is said that all of us have circled in these six realms since beginningless time, and that if all the skeletons that we have had in our various lives were heaped up, the pile would exceed the height of Mount Sumeru. If all the mothers' milk that we have drunk throughout our countless existences was collected, the amount would exceed the amount of water in all the oceans. So now that we practise the Dharma, we must do so without delay. [137]

## 28.2  Reaching Rebirth

While consciousness is within the Bardo, it is possible to access that consciousness. Where a shaman has been asked to perform a soul retrieval or help a soul be reborn, this is where and when the shaman will contact the soul. He or she helps consciousness not be afraid, helps them develop a positive mindset, and helps them understand what is happening and what is next in the Bardo.

After a certain amount of time, it can be some seconds, some minutes, some hours, some days. At a maximum of 49 days, the consciousness will arrive at the spot where the rebirth will take place.

If we are to accept the psychology of the Sidpa Bardo, it is characterized by the fierce wind of karma, which whirls the dead man along until he comes to the "womb-door." The Sidpa state permits no going back, because it is sealed off against the Chonyid [Bardo] state by an intense striving downwards, towards the animal sphere of instinct and physical rebirth. [138]

According to the state of rebirth, leaving the Bardo and entering that realm will be slightly different. For example, if you are to take birth in the god realm, you are not going through a development

---

[135] Ibid.

[136] Dharmakaya, "Dharmakaya Buddhist Concept."

[137] https://www.budsas.org/ebud/whatbudbeliev/96.htm, "What Buddhists Believe - Rebirth."

[138] https://carljungdepthpsychologysite.blog/2019/04/29/carl-jung-on-the-tibetan-book-of-the-dead/#.Xmt2-qrX23A, "Carl Jung on the Tibetan Book of the Dead – Carl Jung Depth Psychology."

process like an embryo would develop in a womb—it's a spontaneous birth. The process is slightly different also if you take rebirth as a spirit or a ghost or in a Hell realm—it will also be a spontaneous rebirth. Only in the animal realm or in the human realm it will be a period of gestation.

When the soul, the consciousness reaches this point at which the soul, as described in the Bardo Thodol, ends with rebirth in the womb.[139]

---

[139] Ibid.

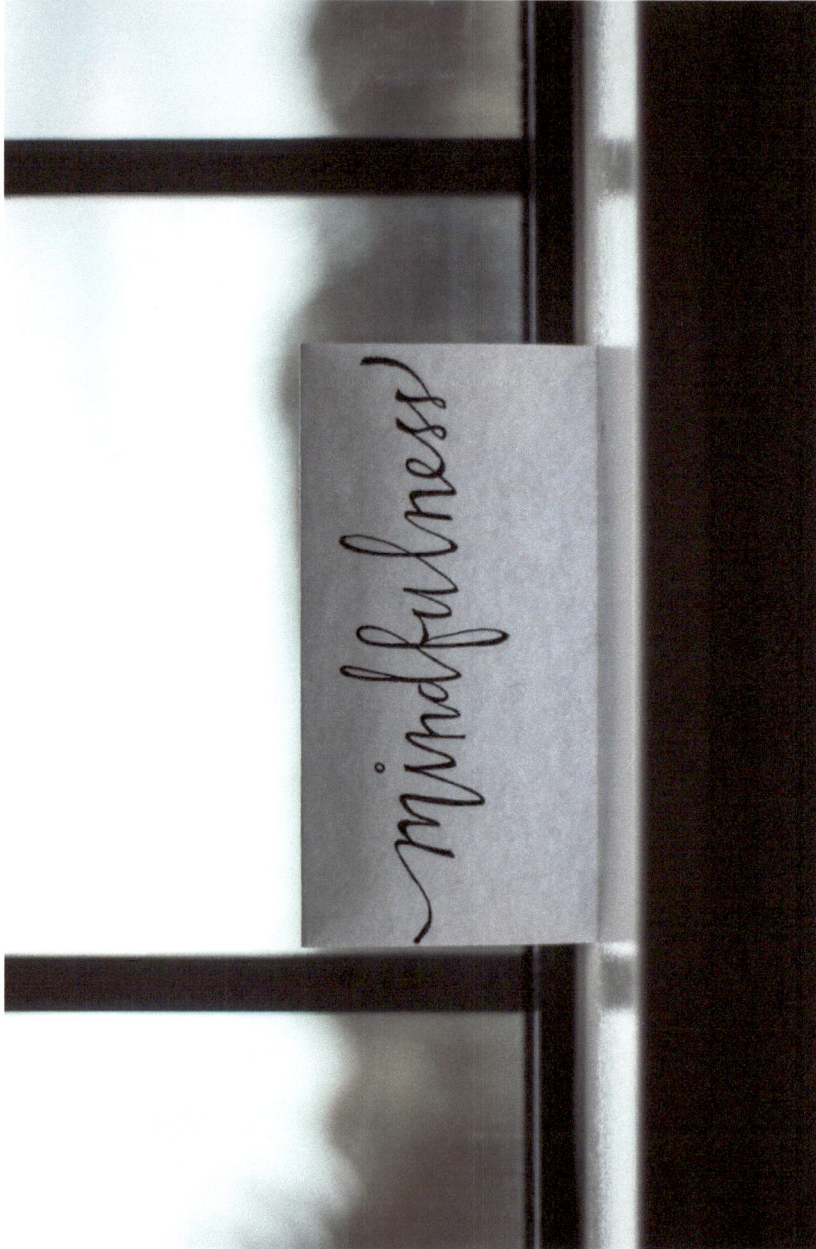

*Figure 4. Be Mindful. Photo by Lesly Juarez on Unsplash*

*Figure 5. Be mindful*

## 29  Mindfulness

**M**indfulness is the practice of being fully present in the moment. If we are looking at a flower, our attention is fully engrossed, consumed, by the flower and our experience from looking at the flower and all that is around us at that moment. Our mind does not wander to anything else.

Unfortunately, this is not always the case. Research by psychologists Matthew A. Killingsworth and Daniel T. Gilbert at Harvard University has discovered that people spend 46.9% of their waking hours thinking about something other than what they're doing, and this mind-wandering typically makes them unhappy.[140]

Usually, as a person's mind wanders, they end up thinking about the past, the future, events that are happening, or not now. If it is the past, it might be a breakup of a relationship. Could I have done better? Could I rekindle the relationship? Why did I say that? Why did I literally walk away? These are things that are not in the here and now, and things I cannot change by thinking about it. If it is the future, it is worried over the outcome of an event that has not occurred, and if it is now, at this moment, can you change what is about to happen, or not?

One of the most common results of overthinking or mind wandering and thinking about things we cannot change is unhappiness. Replaying the events of a scenario, and devising alternative outcomes, which didn't happen, is exhausting and spirals into further mind wandering, stress, and unhappiness.

Meditation is a practice that helps us understand and practise mindfulness and being in the present and not where the busy mind wants to take us. The most common tool in meditation and mindfulness is concentration on breathing. It is the simplest tool that comes with our physical human state. Breathing on and out and then graduating to being able to breathe in through one nostril and out through the other. This takes practice, but like any skill, what we practise becomes natural to us and easier until we do it without thinking.

When our mind wanders and creates worry, stress, anxiety, and judgment, we strengthen those emotions and habits. We are strengthening the mental pathways that create those scenarios and results. It is like a drug. The more we worry, the stronger those habits become so that we can "enjoy" them all over again. Scientifically, this is called neuroplasticity[141] [142] by repetition the brain develops and parts of it become thicker, richer, and more capable, by what we understand now as cortical thickening. Meditation is a habit that has been identified to grow bigger brains.[143] In one area of grey matter, the thickening turns out to be more pronounced in older than in younger people. That's intriguing because those sections of the human cortex, or thinking cap, normally get thinner as we age.[144]

---

[140] https://news.harvard.edu/gazette/story/2010/11/wandering-mind-not-a-happy-mind/, "Wandering Mind Not a Happy Mind."

[141141] https://en.wikipedia.org/wiki/Neuroplasticity, "Neuroplasticity."

[142] https://www.sciencedirect.com/topics/medicine-and-dentistry/neural-plasticity, "Neural Plasticity."

[143] https://news.harvard.edu/gazette/story/2006/02/meditation-found-to-increase-brain-size/, "Meditation Found to Increase Brain Size."

[144] Ibid.

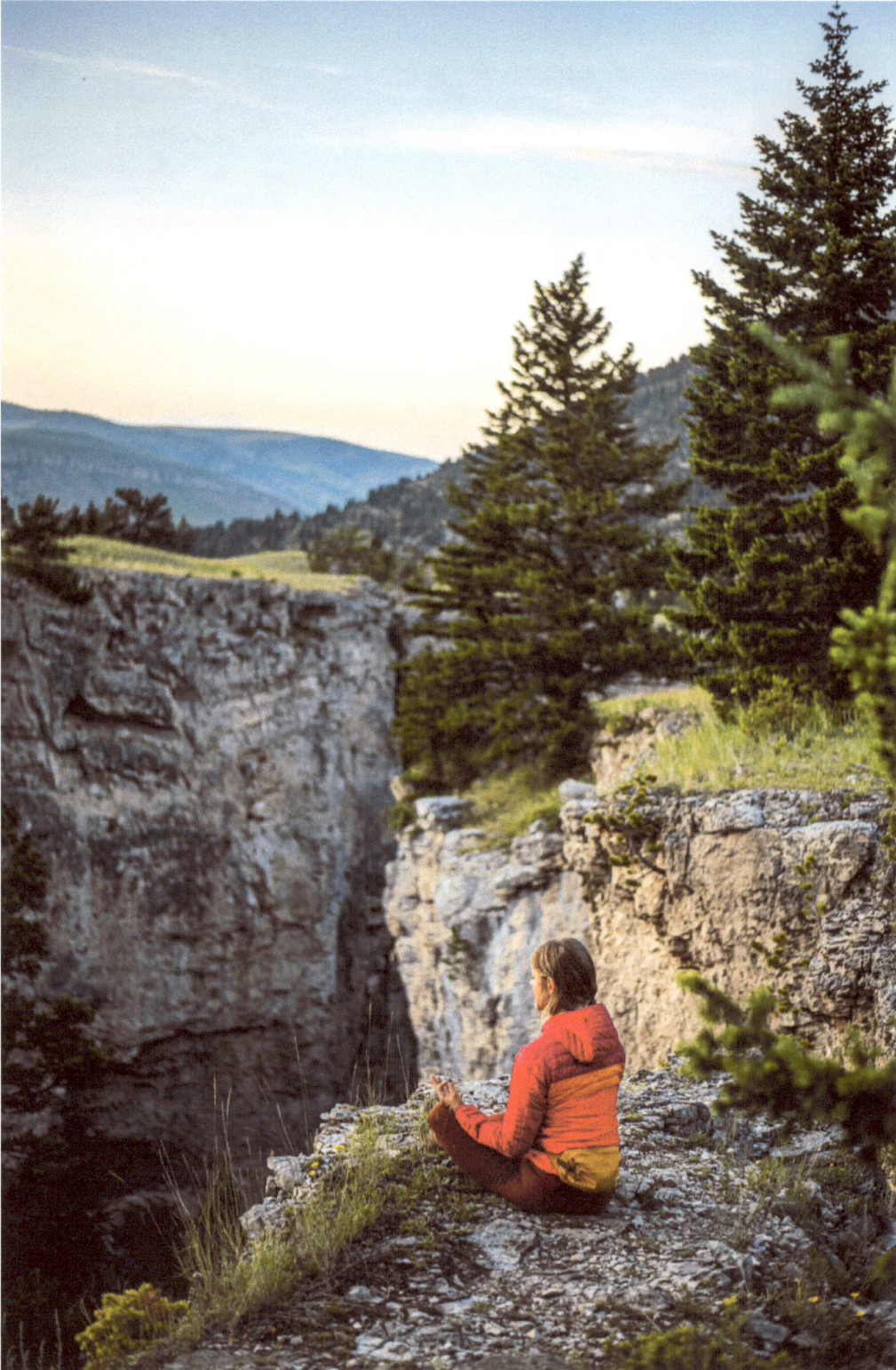

*Figure 6. Meditating in Nature. Photo by Steven Cordes on Unsplash*

## 30   Bardo

In some schools of Buddhism, Bardo is an intermediate, or liminal state between death and rebirth—reincarnation. Reincarnation into another life, as a different being, is the philosophical or religious concept that the non-physical essence of a living being starts a new life in a different physical form or body after biological death. It is also called rebirth or transmigration.[145]

Bardo is a concept which arose soon after the Buddha's passing, with several earlier Buddhist groups accepting the existence of such an intermediate state, while other schools rejected it.

In Tibetan Buddhism, Bardo is the central theme of the Bardo Thodol[146]; literally Liberation Through Hearing During the Intermediate State, in the west, Bardo Thodol is known as the Tibetan Book of the Dead.[147] The Tibetan Book of the Dead is a Lamist book of counsel, probably influenced by Bon shamanism. The Buddhist lama who whispers this sacred text into the dead man's ear is himself, like the tribal shaman, a psychopomp or soul-guide who accompanies the dead person on his difficult path during the forty-nine days of the intermediate state between death and rebirth.[148]

According to Sogyal Rinpoche, death is not something to be feared as a tragedy, but is an opportunity for transformation. In Tibetan tradition, after death and before one's next birth, when one's consciousness is not connected with a physical body, one experiences a variety of phenomena. These usually follow a particular sequence of degeneration from just after death, the clearest experiences of reality of which one is spiritually capable, and then proceeding to terrifying hallucinations that arise from the impulses of one's previous unskillful actions. For the prepared and appropriately trained individuals, the Bardo offers a state of great opportunity for liberation, since transcendental insight may arise with the direct experience of reality; for others, it can become a place of danger, as the karmically created hallucinations can impel one into a less than desirable rebirth.[149]

Symbolically, Bardo can describe times when our usual way of life becomes suspended, as, for example, during a period of illness or during a meditation retreat. Such times can prove fruitful for spiritual progress because external constraints diminish. However, they can also present challenges because our less skillful impulses may come to the foreground, just as in the sidpa Bardo.

The concept of antarabhava,[150] an intervening state between death and rebirth, was brought into Buddhism from the Vedic-Upanishadic philosophical tradition, which later developed into Hinduism.

From the records of ancient Buddhist schools, at least six different groups accepted the notion of an intermediate existence: antarabhava the Sarvastivada, Darstantika, Vatsiputriyas, Sammitiya, Purvasaila and late Mahisasaka. The first four are closely related schools. Opposing them was the Mahasamghika, early Mahisasaka, Theravada, Vibhajyavada and the Sariputra Abhidharma.

---

[145] https://en.wikipedia.org/wiki/The_City_of_God, "The City of God."
[146] Britannica, "Bardo ThöDol Tibetan Buddhist Text."
[147] Wikipedia, "Bardo."
[148] University of California Press eBook Collection, "The Spiritual Quest," (1982 - 2004).
[149] Wikipedia, "Bardo."
[150] https://www.wisdomlib.org, "Antarabhava, AntarāBhava 2 Definitions."

After death, the shaman will undertake a journey to the intermediate world and with their guides and helping spirits seek the soul of the deceased and guide and encourage it to cross over fully, especially if the wandering soul has been affecting the lives of the remaining living relatives or otherwise causing problems.

The shaman may also be asked to help souls and spirits cross over who had no connection to the living but have connected themselves to the living and causing illness.

Battles and confrontations with evil or dark spirits and souls may help a sick individual or help the spirt cross over. The shaman's universe includes an upper, middle, and lower realm where spirits exist, along with the spirits of ancestors who must be understood and persuaded to help a soul in its current physical incarnation.

Because of the split and downright antagonism that often exists between those trained in science and those professing particular religions, there is often little study of each other's accounts of religious and psychic phenomena, so books like those mentioned are often not known outside a narrow circle of experts or academic authorities. Yet Carol Zaleski's book has already spawned a whole academic field of research into the phenomenology of "otherworldly realities"—there have been several international conferences to date—while Sogyal's book is now used worldwide to help people who are nearing death prepare for their passing over. [151]

My first realization[152] of how important it is to follow a person's consciousness into other realms, in whatever way possible, came twenty years ago during a psychotherapy session with a woman who had survived a major car accident and had gone through a classic NDE during subsequent surgery to save her life. She was still suffering from manifest PTSD symptoms when she consulted me and I regressed her to the memory of the accident. Not only did she relive the accident and release much buried trauma held in her body but she also proceeded to re-play the experience of watching herself from above as ambulance men pulled her body from the wreckage. She then saw her body taken to the hospital and undergoing surgery. Next, she felt herself drifting up to a higher realm and meeting with beings of light she recognized as deceased members of her family, who told her that her work on earth was not finished and that she must return. She remembered the pain of coming back into her body. Prior to the regression, she had not "remembered" any of this. The session profoundly altered her attitude to death and dying. Indeed, what most deeply struck her was the continuity of her consciousness both before and after her "death" and both in and out of her body.[153]

In Buddhism, some of the earliest references we have the "intermediate existence" are found in the Sarvastivadin text the Mahavibhasa. For instance, the Mahavibhasa shows a "basic existence," an "intermediate existence," a "birth existence" and "death existence."

The intermediate being who makes the passage in this way from one existence to the next is formed, like every living being, of the five aggregate skandhas[154]. Existence is shown because it cannot have any discontinuity in time and space between the place and moment of death and those of rebirth, and therefore it must be that the two existences belonging to the same series are linked in time and space by an intermediate stage. The intermediate being is the Gandharva, which

[151] Dr. Roger J. Woolger, "Beyond Death- Transition and the Afterlife."
[152] Ibid.
[153] Ibid.
[154] Wikipedia, "Skandha."

is as necessary for conception as the fecundity and union of the parents. The Antaraparinirvayin is an Anagamin who gets parinirvana during the intermediary existence. As for the heinous criminal guilty of one of the five crimes without interval (Anantara), he passes in quite the same way by an intermediate existence at the end of which he is reborn, necessarily in hell.[155]

What is an intermediate being and an intermediate existence? Intermediate existence, which inserts itself between existence at death and existence at birth, not having arrived at the location where it should go, cannot be said to be born. Between death, the five skandhas of the moment of death—and arising, the five skandhas of the moment of rebirth—there is found an existence—a "body" of five skandhas—that goes to the place of rebirth. This existence between two realms of rebirth (gati) is called an intermediate existence.

He cites several texts and examples to defend the notion against other schools, which reject it and claim that death in one life is immediately followed by rebirth in the next, with no intermediate state in between the two. Both the Mahavibhasa and the Abhidharmakosa have the notion of the intermediate state lasting "seven times seven days" i.e., 49 days at most. This is one view, though, and there were also others.[156]

## 30.1  Bardo States

These are transitional states within the 49-day period the soul of the deceased is transitioning to their next life, their rebirth. But Bardo refers to that state in which we have lost our old reality and it is no longer available to us.

What makes death and impermanence so painful is our idea of the strict dichotomy between existence and nonexistence. Knowing something beyond that dualism is paramount. At the moment of death, instead of being caught between the ideas of existence and nonexistence, instead of this crisis of having everything that matters to us taken away all at once, something else can open up entirely; we shift our attention to the nucleus of being, to present itself and experiencing itself.[157]

Without some way of managing this experience, this unsettling discontinuity punctuated by occasional disruptions to the very idea of our being, we never know if we are going to show up in the next moment as a Buddha or as a demon. We're like gods one moment, tasting the fruit of the kingdom, and hungry ghosts the next, not even able to swallow it. How confusing—and how fantastic! This confusion is the raw material of wisdom. Our path is to find a presence in each of these experiences. In the Bardo case, when presence is the only real thing left, if we are searching for security instead, wisdom can be elusive. It's no wonder that religion becomes so poignant during times of crisis; suddenly, presence is all we are. Everything else recedes except what is right in front of us. Recognizing this opens up the potential to experience life with awareness of impermanence and the presence it illuminates.[158]

---

[155] "Bardo."
[156] Ibid.
[157] Lionsroar.com, "The Four Points of Letting Go in the Bardo."
[158] Ibid.

- Rupture: There is a total rupture in our who-I-am, and we are forced to undergo a great and difficult transformation.

This is the Vajrayana awareness of successive deaths and rebirths, and it is the first essential point to understand: rupture. The more we learn to recognize this sense of disruption, the more willing and able we will be to let go of this notion of an inherent reality and allow that precious pot to slip out of our hands. Rupture takes place all the time, day to day and moment to moment; in fact, as soon as we see our life in terms of these successive deaths and rebirths, we dissolve the very idea of a solid self-grasping onto an inherently real life. We start to see how conditional who-I-am-ness really is and how even that does not provide reliable ground upon which to stand.

- Emptying the Contrived Self:

This is shunyata[159], which gets translated in various ways, most commonly as "emptiness," but there is no real correlation in our language, no single word or idea that can cover this ground of disrupted reality. Because "emptiness" in English has negative connotations, shunyata is sometimes translated as "voidness," "open spaciousness," and even "boundlessness"; Angoumois[160] such as Longchenpa explained emptiness in positive terms inextricably associated with presence, clarity, and compassion. But in death and birth, shunyata refers to a direct experience of disruption felt at the core of our being when there is no longer any use manufacturing artificial security.[161]

- Recognize that our experience is based on dynamic, responsive presence.

Our goal is to learn to relax and how to do so and to fall into the inherent peacefulness of not knowing what comes next. When we do—and if we do—everything changes. We are no longer slaves to primordial anxiety.

Experiencing a loss can be freeing. When we are free of all our psychological heaviness and the accumulated weight of our usual momentum, we know the raw presence that remains. To be a Buddhist is to dedicate our lives to abiding in that impermanent, empty, visceral presence. We can bear with greater ease those losses that we know we will inevitably face because we identify with the thread of wakefulness that we meet in all of them. And then perhaps, when death draws near, we can relax with ease into the ground of being as we shed this skin, finally let go of this body, and experience liberation—undefended being in groundless space.[162]

## 30.2  The Six Bardos in Tibetan Buddhism

The Bardo Thodol differentiates the intermediate state between lives into three bardos:

1. Kyenay Bardo/Shinay Bardo (Tibetan)—Skye gnas bar does is the first Bardo of birth and life. This Bardo begins from conception until the last breath when the mind stream withdraws from the body.

---

[159] www.rigpawiki.org, "Emptiness."
[160] "Nyingma Buddhism."
[161] Lionsroar.com, "The Four Points of Letting Go in the Bardo."
[162] Ibid.

2. Milam Bardo—rmi lam bar does is the second Bardo of the dream state. The Milam Bardo is a subset of the first Bardo. Dream Yoga develops practices to integrate the dream state into Buddhist Sadhana.

3. Samten Bardo—bsam gtan bar does is the third Bardo of meditation. This Bardo is only experienced by meditators, though individuals may have spontaneous experience of it. Samten Bardo is a subset of the Shinay Bardo.

4. Chikhai Bardo—'chi kha'i bar does is the fourth Bardo of the moment of death. According to tradition, this Bardo is held to begin when the outer and inner signs presage that the onset of death is nigh, and continue through the dissolution or transmutation of the Mahabhuta until the external and internal breath has completed.

*This is the first of three intermediate states between lives in the Tibetan Book of the dead.*

5. Chonyid Bardo—whose nyid bar does, is the fifth Bardo of the luminosity of true nature, which begins after the final "inner breath" Sanskrit: prana, Vayu; Tibetan: rlung. It is within this Bardo that visions and auditory phenomena occur. In the Dzogchen teachings, these are known as the spontaneously manifesting Thodgal Tibetan: thod-rgyal visions.

Connected to these visions, there is a welling of profound peace and pristine awareness. Sentient beings who have not practised during their lived experience and/or who do not recognize the clear light Tibetan: OD gsal at the moment of death is usually deluded throughout the fifth Bardo of luminosity.

*This is the second of three intermediate states between lives in the Tibetan Book of the dead.*

6. Sidpa Bardo—srid pay bar does is the sixth Bardo of becoming or transmigration. This Bardo endures until the inner breath begins in the new transmigrating form determined by the "karmic seeds" within the storehouse consciousness.

*This is the third of three intermediate states between lives in the Tibetan Book of the dead.*

## 30.3  The Liberation Through Hearing During the Intermediate State

C. G. Jung's[163] psychological commentary on the Tibetan Book of the Dead first appeared in an English translation by R. F. C. Hull in the third revised and expanded Evans-Wentz edition of The Tibetan Book of the Dead.

He does not attempt to directly correlate the content of the Bardo Thodol with rituals or dogma found in occidental religion, but highlights karmic phenomena described on the Bardo plane and shows how they parallel unconscious contents both personal and collective encountered in the west, particularly in analytical psychology. [164]

---

[163] Wikipedia, "Carl Jung."
[164] "Bardo Thodol."

Jung's comments should be taken strictly within the realm of psychology, and not that of theology or metaphysics. Indeed, he repeatedly warns of the dangers for western man in the wholesale adoption of eastern religious traditions, such as yoga. [165]

1. "Life," or ordinary waking consciousness;

2. "Dhyana" (meditation);

   In the oldest texts of Buddhism, dhyāna (Sanskrit) or jhāna (Pali) is the training of the mind, commonly translated as meditation, to withdraw the mind from the automatic responses to sense impressions, leading to a "state of perfect equanimity and awareness (upekkhā-sati-parisuddhi)." Dhyana may have been the core practice of pre-sectarian Buddhism, in combination with several related practices, which together lead to perfected mindfulness and detachment, and are fully realized with the practice of dhyana.

3. "Dream," the dream state during normal sleep.

Together these "six bardos" form a classification of states of consciousness into six broad types. Any state of consciousness can form a type of "intermediate state," intermediate between other states of consciousness.[166]

---

[165] Ibid.
[166] Ibid.

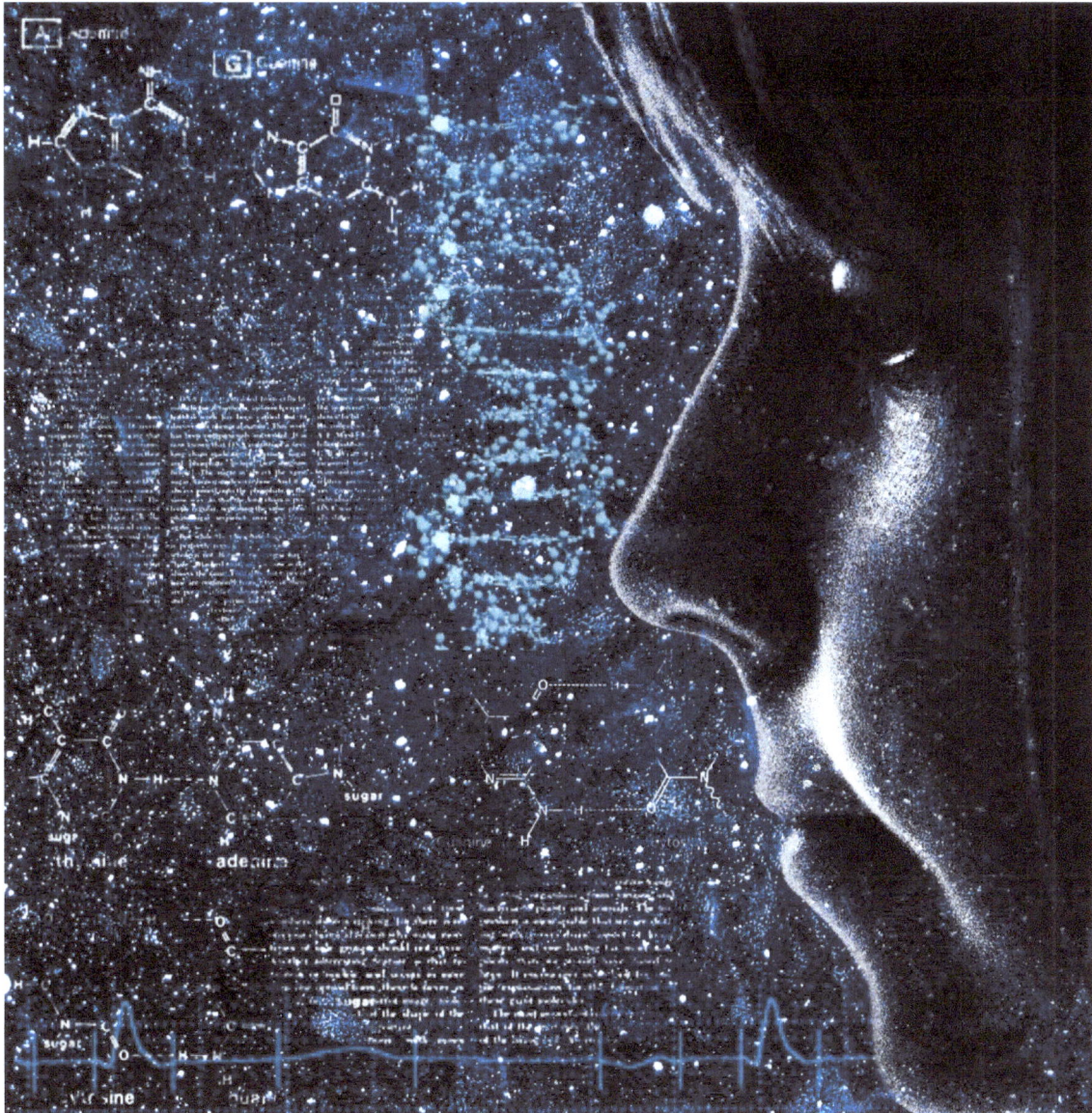

*Figure 7. Looking at Evolution*

## 31   Karmic Evolution

**Y**ou incarnate to advance both your individual wisdom and collective wisdom. Moving through your lifetimes to greater light, you advance from incarnations primarily centred on your own soul progress to lives that serve the progress of humanity. The knowledge that you achieve through each lifetime benefits not only you as an individual soul; your trials and tribulations also enhance the greater whole of humanity and the universe. Your intrinsic reason for incarnating gradually becomes easier and easier to discern. You discover you are here to be of service. Eventually, you reach a level of development where you serve as a teacher or guide for other souls. This is sometimes referred to as "Ascension."[167]

As we move through different lives, facing unique challenges, suffering, and benefits, the worlds into which we incarnate are changing. Darwinian evolution describes what has taken place over very long periods of time.

Darwin's finches on the Galapagos Islands did not develop the differences in their beaks and their feeding habits in one lifetime. The lifespan of a finch is 7 years and can be as short as 4 years. It took a lot longer than that to make the evolutionary change that results in a different beak shape.

Vaster periods of history are required to change behaviour and physical characteristics. A cave dweller is a stock character representative of primitive man in the Paleolithic. The Paleolithic, also called the Old Stone Age, is a period in human prehistory distinguished by the original development of stone tools that cover c. 99% of the time of human technological prehistory. It extends from the earliest known use of stone tools by hominin c. 3.3 million years ago, to the end of the Pleistocene c. 11,650 cal BP.[168] The popularization of the type dates to the early 20th century, when Neanderthal Man was influentially described as "simian" or apelike by Marcellin Boule and Arthur Keith.[169]

While knowledge of human evolution in the Pleistocene has become much more detailed, the stock character has not disappeared, even though it anachronistically conflates characteristics of archaic and early modern humans.

So, from cave dwellers to today [2020], it is well over 3 million years. Even with humans' ability to gain knowledge, use tools, and to learn rapidly, that is still a long period.

Humanity has intervened intentionally or unintentionally in virtually all aspects of physical existence on this planet. Humanity has changed the way animals live and sometimes suffer. Some would argue that Karma cannot influence the rebirth of a soul into a physical container called a "body" or "Host" so that the soul can learn aspects of spiritual existence it needs.

But soul and container are symbiotically linked. The soul experiences existence within the confines of the physical container, the body. The body imposes restrictions or provides advantages through its ability to function in certain ways. These restrictions or advantages may be openly apparent. Some may not be apparent until some form of interaction comes to light. For example, deafness, or being "hard of hearing."

---

[167] https://www.ravenheartcenter.com/index.php/soul-evolution, "Soul Evolution Clear Past Life Karma and Live Your Life Purpose."
[168] Wikipedia, "Paleolithic."
[169] "Caveman."

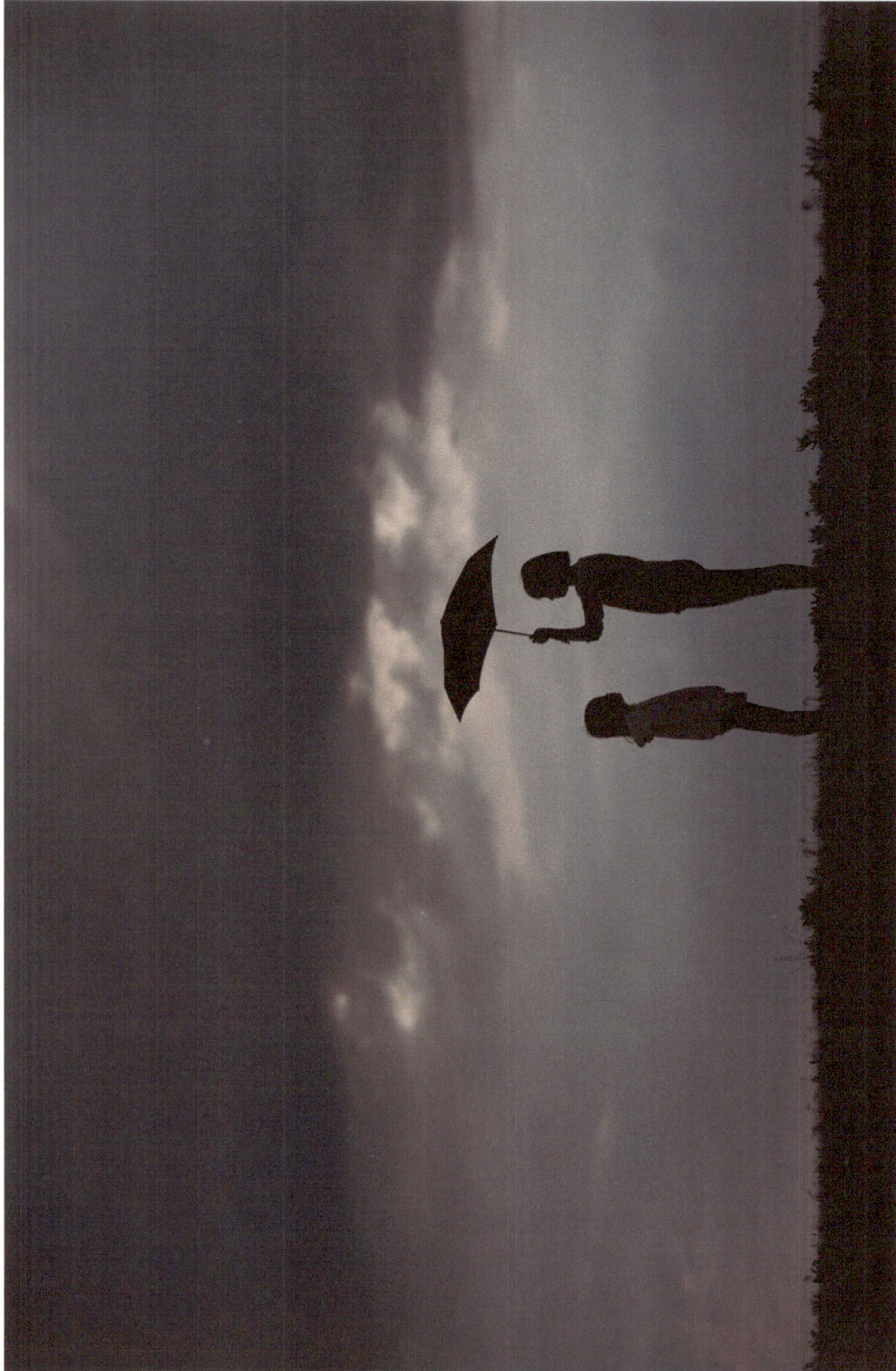

*Figure 8. Help. Photo by J W on Unsplash*

## 32   Deafness

For many years growing up, I lived next to a family whose son was described as hard of hearing. From a karmic view, his soul had been reincarnated into a container, a physical form, a body with a hearing defect that would, throughout his life, confront him with innumerable challenges. Loving parents, doctors, and educators in our modern society worked tirelessly to help overcome these challenges and provide as natural a life as possible growing up.

We think of Karma in terms of the soul that is being reincarnated, but we need to consider those around and intimately linked to the reincarnated soul. Their reincarnation may seem clear of worry, but the simple act of a challenged child, or an aged parent, has affected that affects subsequent reincarnation of souls of all those connected. It is a clear representation of the fact that we are all interconnected.

It was not just the person I played with as I grew up that was affected. His parents were challenged by the need to care for him, teach him and struggle to ensure what he was entitled to from the education and medical systems was delivered not just once, but regularly.

Deaf people may have no trouble communicating any ideas in American Sign Language, or ASL, that can be expressed in English. But studies of ASL signers show that, on average, deaf high school seniors are likely to read at the level of a nine-year-old. The explanation has always been that this is because they never learned to connect letters with sounds. But a recent study shows that deaf readers are just like other people learning to read in a second language.[170]

The assumption has always been that the problems with reading were educational issues with what's the right way to teach reading when you can't associate sounds with letters. But what we're finding is that all this time we've been ignoring the fact that they're actually learning a new language. Jill Morford. [171]

Ms. Morford is a professor at the University of New Mexico and part of a research centre at Gallaudet University in Washington. Most students at Gallaudet are deaf; the centre studies how deaf people learn and use language. [172]

Professor Morford says signers are like English learners whose first language uses a different alphabet.

Anyone who has a first language that has a written system that's very different from English, like Arabic or Chinese or Russian, knows that learning to recognize and understand words in English is much more challenging than if you already speak a language that uses the same orthography. [173]

Gallaudet Professor Tom Allen explains what effect this has on reading. We're not dealing with representations in the brain which are primarily auditory. You know, people when they read, they hear—there's a silent hearing going on when you read a word, when a hearing person reads a word. When a deaf person reads a word, there's not. They see the word and there's some kind of

---

[170] https://learningenglish.voanews.com/a/a-new-reason-for-why-the-deaf-may-have-trouble-reading-119728279/115194.html, "A New Reason for Why the Deaf May Have Trouble Reading."
[171] Ibid.
[172] Ibid.
[173] Ibid.

orthographic representation. And some of the research in our centre has shown that when deaf readers read an English word, it activates their sign representations of those words.[174]

As policies towards the hard of hearing changed, my friend's parents had to keep pace with the changes and decide for his, and they, own best interest. In terms of their working lives, this was an added burden that any parent with a child who faces some type of challenge will sympathize with and understand.

They also had to deal with the sometimes hidden, or not hidden mentality that to have a child with a disability reflected on the father, and, or, the mother's ability to produce a healthy offspring. A genuine issue in olden times when there were abundant challenges in the world without being thought of as fathering or delivering children that could not participate fully in society.

The souls of his parents reincarnated twenty or thirty years prior to his birth, but they were equally challenged. The simple difference between "Hard of Hearing" and the word "deaf" was not just about the difference in terminology but about the linkage of deaf with disabilities.

Disability is linked to "cannot do" or "cannot perform," with the emphasis on "cannot." When it came time for me to get a weekend job to earn some pocket money rather than take an allowance from my parents, I chose a retail setting where I am interacting with customers. That choice was not open to him because shop managers had the mindset that deaf people are difficult to work with, or cannot follow instructions, or cannot interact with customers properly because they do not articulate. He got a weekend job, but it was a "back of the store" role where he was moving stock around, or filling shelves.

It paid less and denied him the wide and diverse range of human interaction that I benefited from. It also linked his expectations and feelings about himself, his value in society and what he could achieve with this lower paid, more menial work.

The first hearing aid was created in the 17th century. The movement towards modern hearing aids began with the creation of the telephone, and the first electric hearing aid was created in 1898. The first electronic hearing aids were constructed after the invention of the telephone and microphone in the 1870s and 1880s. The technology within the telephone increased how acoustic signals could be altered. Telephones could control the loudness, frequency, and distortion of sounds. These abilities were used in the hearing's creation aid. By the late 20th century, the digital hearing aid was distributed to the public commercially. Some of the first hearing aids were external hearing aids. External hearing aids directed sounds in front of the ear and blocked all other noises. The apparatus would fit behind or in the ear. [175]

Our understanding of deafness and hearing loss differs vastly from someone from those earlier periods. A soul born into a body with a hearing defect in the 17th century would have differed vastly from the same soul being reincarnated into a body with the same defect today—2020.

---

[174] Ibid.
[175] Wikipedia, "History of Hearing Aids."

Today we understand hearing defects and loss as being described as: Cross-Modal Cortical Reorganization [176] [177]

The brain is the centre of operations for our entire body, but it can be affected by both physical and intangible ailments. While hearing loss affects our ability to hear, it can also lead to changes in the brain. [178]

Hearing loss can occur in anyone, no matter their age or race. Because hearing loss affects so many aspects of people's lives, there have been many studies to explore how it changes the brain. The results are interesting and show how much the brain can alter to make up for lost senses. Neuroplasticity refers to the rewiring of the brain to handle new functions and situations. In people with hearing loss, the brain is rewired in several ways. [179]

Despite the long name, this is actually not a complicated process. When hearing loss occurs, the brain has to overcompensate for this lost sense. By placing additional emphasis on other senses, like touch and vision, this process leads to fatigue and adversely affects concentration. [180]

While this can help hard-of-hearing people cope with the loss of their hearing, it can cause detrimental effects to brain function. For example, when a person experiences hearing loss, the area of the brain that processes sound begins to deteriorate. This leads to problems understanding speech and language. Because the brain has to overcompensate for these weakening brain functions, higher-level thinking is forfeited for speech understanding.

This can lead to a host of other problems, including the possible acceleration of dementia.

People who are hearing impaired experience and navigate the world much differently than those with perfect hearing. To gain an understanding of the difficulties they may face, here are ten situations you may have never thought of that make life more challenging when little to nothing is audible.

| Challenge | Meaning |
|---|---|
| Public announcements | Public address systems notify us of what's going on all the time, but a hearing-impaired individual probably won't get the message. |
| Slow talkers | When someone realizes they're interacting with a hearing-impaired person, they often switch to a slower form of speech. While it's done with the best intentions, it can actually hinder lip reading. Over time, the hearing impaired have learned to understand words when people speak naturally, so slowing it down intentionally can cause miscommunication. |
| Being in the Dark | Whether it's a dimly lit room or a noisy dark club, the absence of light makes it difficult for the hearing impaired to engage with others. They rely on visual stimuli, such as lip-reading or sign language, so darkness poses a challenge. |
| Being "jumpy" | Have you ever been startled by someone approaching you from behind? It happens to the hearing impaired all the time. Without visual cues or vibrations on the floor, they can be easily startled. For some, this leads to a constant "jumpy" |

---

[176] https://www.britannica.com/science/cross-modal-plasticity, "Cross-Modal Plasticity Biology Britannica."
[177] https://www.signia-hearing.com/blog/how-does-hearing-loss-affect-the-brain/, "How Hearing Loss Affects the Brain and Associated Risks - Signia Hearing Aids."
[178] Ibid.
[179] Ibid.
[180] Ibid.

| Challenge | Meaning |
|---|---|
| | feeling, as they can rarely be completely comfortable. No one is sneaking up on them from behind. |
| Relying on Touch | When most of us want someone's attention, we can simply call out their name. When a person is hearing impaired, however, they won't hear their name called. That's why in deaf culture, firm but polite tapping on the shoulder is normal in order to gain attention. However, those not familiar with the deaf community may be unaware of this, leading to confrontation. |
| Sign Language Misunderstandings | Sign language is far from universal, and different standards exist in different countries (for example, the differences between American and British Sign Language are quite significant). In addition, regional areas have their own specific variations—just like accents or slang—leading to further difficulty. There are many instances of professional interpreters using the wrong words because of the variations across regions and countries; while this may not seem like a big deal, it has led to lasting harm, such as in legal situations or miscommunication during hospital visits. |
| Job Applications and Interviews | Job interviews are already stressful situations; now consider being hearing impaired. Those who are hard of hearing or deaf may sometimes feel completely ignored when they reveal their hearing status on application forms, possibly because recruiters see it as too much extra work to accommodate them. When they reach the interview stage, more complications arise. Telephone interviews are nearly impossible without an interpreter, and in-person interviews can be difficult to carry out if an interviewer is unprepared for the situation. |
| Going to a Movie | Seeing the newest films at a theatre is no easy feat. Often, theatre chains are unreliable with setting up films with subtitles; if they have subtitled films available, they're often only on films that have been out for months or shown at unusual times, such as 10 a.m. on a Wednesday. |
| Caring for Hearing Aids | While hearing aids have helped millions to better hear sounds and communicate more effectively with others, they also have to be well maintained to keep the equipment working optimally. The hearing impaired often have to keep spare batteries when travelling or commuting, and because the devices can't get wet, even a midafternoon rainstorm can pose a problem. |
| Depression and Anxiety | Studies reveal deaf people are around twice as likely to suffer from psychological problems such as depression and anxiety. Research suggests this stems from feelings of isolation. Making matters worse, the most effective treatment for these types of issues is usually talking with a therapist. Of course, finding a doctor or therapist with the means necessary to effectively work with those who have hearing challenges is no easy feat. |

*Figure 9. Table taken from "Public address systems notify us of what's going on all the time, but a hearing-impaired individual probably won't get the message."* [181]

The hearing impaired and the deaf have learned to adjust to many situations. There will always be challenges. Thankfully, technology is helping change lives. For example, many public announcements are now also sent to cell phones. While many deaf people don't want hearing and consider deafness their own unique culture, the larger hearing world still views them with pity. The fact is, most deaf people or hearing-impaired individuals don't want pity, but just want to be treated with respect. As hearing individuals, that is the most important thing we can provide. [182]

---

[181] https://www.disabilityexpertsfl.com/blog/difficulties-the-deaf-face-every-day, "Difficulties the Hearing Impaired Face Every Day."
[182] Ibid.

## 33   Darwin, Karma, and the Process of Rebirth

In some schools of Buddhism, Bardo, antarabhava, or chuu is an intermediate or liminal state between death and rebirth—reincarnation. Reincarnation into another life, as a different being, is the philosophical or religious concept that the non-physical essence of a living being starts a new life in a different physical form or body after biological death. It is also called rebirth or transmigration.[183]

The Buddhist view is that a person's actions shape his or her own future existence and ultimately determine into which of the six realms they will take rebirth following death. This means that people who do not believe in God but do-good deeds during their lives will not go to hell. The Buddhist theory of karma holds that you are what you do. Even those who don't believe in the Buddha will reap the rewards in a future life if they do well and avoid all harmful acts. Buddhist karma tells us that positive action results in beneficial reaction, whereas negative action results in unwanted reaction. Therefore, it is often said that karma follows a person like a shadow.[184]

It is important to remember that when the soul consciousness leaves the physical body, it may remain for a while around the body, in a favourite room, or around a favourite person without connecting to the dead body. When the soul leaves its body, it will see it and not connect with the meaning of it. This sets it apart from the Out of Body Experiences, where there is a connection, a necessary connection to what is still a physically living body.

The connection of the soul disappeared in the dissolution stage of dying. However, death is usually a very emotional environment. People are crying, expressing themselves emotionally, naming the body, recalling his life and his qualities, his virtues, etc. Maybe competitors or people who did not like him are criticizing, complaining, and glad that he is no longer physically around. But all of this, the good and the bad, are gone. Dissolution has restarted the counter: the memories of consciousness. A Shaman will be called if the emotions of those who knew the soul in physical form are so strong, they hold the soul to the physical realm, causing reconnection with them. Later, if the soul disconnects but does not complete the process of rebirth, it may wander the physical realm, connecting to people with which it has no purpose, but sometimes injury those living souls and consciousness.

### 33.1   Is Rebirth Simultaneous?

A controversial subject I rebirth is whether it is simultaneous with death. According to Abhidhamma, rebirth or conception, as it is known, takes place immediately after the death of a being with no intermediate state. Some others believe that a person, after his death, would develop into a spirit form for a certain number of days before rebirth takes place. Another interpretation regarding the same belief is that it is not the spirit, but the deceased person's consciousness or mental energy remaining in space, supported by his own mental energies of craving and attachment. However, eventually rebirth must take place. The spirit petas, who are beings born in spirit form, are unfortunately living beings and their lives in the spirit form are not permanent. It is also rebirth which is temporary.[185]

---

[183] https://en.wikipedia.org/wiki/The_City_of_God, "The City of God."

[184] https://link.springer.com/article/10.1186/s40613-015-0016-2, "On the Naturalization of Karma and Rebirth."

[185] https://www.budsas.org/ebud/whatbudbeliev/96.htm, "What Buddhists Believe - Rebirth."

A concept many people have difficulty with is that, in the process of rebirth, a human being may be reborn as an animal and an animal may be reborn as a human being. The animal nature of the mind and the animal way of life adopted by him can cause him to be reborn as an animal. The condition and behaviour of the mind handle the next existence. A person who is born in animal form, owing to certain mental abuses during a previous birth, could be reborn as a human being if that animal has committed none serious evil acts. Some animals are very intelligent and understanding. This is clear evidence to prove that they are tending towards a human life. A person who is reborn as an animal can again be born as a human being when the bad karma which conditioned his birth as an animal is spent and the good karma which was stored. [186]

It is foolish to waste human existence along with the conducive conditions that we enjoy in free societies and the opportunity that we have to practise the Dharma[187]. It is extremely important that having this opportunity we make use of it. If we cannot practise the Dharma in this life, there is no way of knowing where in the six realms we will be reborn, and when we shall have such a chance again. We must strive to free ourselves from the cycle of rebirth because failing to do so means that we will continue to circle endlessly among these six realms of existence. When the karma, wholesome or unwholesome, that causes us to be born in any of the six realms is exhausted, rebirth will occur, and we will find ourselves again in another realm. In fact, it is said that all of us have circled in these six realms since beginningless time, and that if all the skeletons that we have had in our various lives were heaped up, the pile would exceed the height of Mount Sumeru. If all the mothers' milk that we have drunk throughout our countless existences was collected, the amount would exceed the amount of water in all the oceans. So now that we practise the Dharma, we must do so without delay. [188]

## 33.2  Reaching Rebirth

While consciousness is within the Bardo, it is possible to access that consciousness. Where a shaman has been asked to perform a soul retrieval or help a soul be reborn, this is where and when the shaman will contact the soul. He or she helps consciousness not be afraid, helps them develop a positive mindset, and helps them understand what is happening and what is next in the Bardo.

After a certain amount of time, it can be some seconds, some minutes, some hours, some days. At a maximum of 49 days, the consciousness will arrive at the spot where the rebirth will take place.

If we are to accept the psychology of the Sidpa Bardo, it is characterized by the fierce wind of karma, which whirls the dead man along until he comes to the "womb-door." The Sidpa state permits no going back, because it is sealed off against the Chonyid [Bardo] state by an intense striving downwards, towards the animal sphere of instinct and physical rebirth. [189]

According to the state of rebirth, leaving the Bardo and entering that realm will be slightly different. For example, if you are to take birth in the god realm, you are not going through a development process like an embryo would develop in a womb—it's a spontaneous birth. The process is slightly

---

[186] Ibid.

[187] Dharmakaya, "Dharmakaya Buddhist Concept."

[188] https://www.budsas.org/ebud/whatbudbeliev/96.htm, "What Buddhists Believe - Rebirth."

[189] https://carljungdepthpsychologysite.blog/2019/04/29/carl-jung-on-the-tibetan-book-of-the-dead/#.Xmt2-qrX23A, "Carl Jung on the Tibetan Book of the Dead – Carl Jung Depth Psychology."

different also if you take rebirth as a spirit or a ghost or in a Hell realm—it will also be a spontaneous rebirth. Only in the animal realm or in the human realm it will be a period of gestation.

When the soul, the consciousness reaches this point at which the soul, as described in the Bardo Thodol, ends with rebirth in the womb.[190]

## 33.3  Darwinian Evolution

Darwinian evolution is adapting and changing physical containers, what we perceive as the body and environment in which man and animals exist and in which souls reincarnate. It may not be apparent to us because we do not have the long-term view of the survivors and failures of humanity, or the creatures into which souls may be reincarnated. If only Lucy[191] could speak!

We can record the demise of species of animals within a collective human lifetime. Through evolution, species arise through the process of speciation—where new varieties of organisms arise and thrive when they can find and exploit an ecological niche—and species become extinct when they can no longer survive in changing conditions or against superior competition. The relationship between animals and their ecological niches has been firmly established. A typical species becomes extinct within 10 million years of its first appearance, although some species, called living fossils, survive with little to no morphological change for hundreds of millions of years.[192]

A soul incarnated several hundred years ago would face dramatically different social and physical challenges and outcomes, from today, or a hundred years from now, in the future. But all challenges and outcomes are consistent with the time in which incarnation occurs.

In the classroom of each soul's existence on earth, it is important to see Darwinism as an energetic, if slow-moving force affecting the experiences our spiritual teachers bring us. These teachers are a complex mix of the creators of the stresses we undergo and endure. The situations can adjust duration and intensity of our challenges. They can form the nuances of the challenges, the minor details that can downplay or momentarily force us to our spiritual, and perhaps, physical, knees. They determine the impact on our wider lives and collectively the depth, breadth, and level of our learning.

How you manage these circumstances affects the learning you get from them. Railing in anger and frustration at them is not learning. It is resistance. Ensuring that in the future, the lesson being offered will be re-administered in the future, in a unique form. Being able to do the best you can and see the challenges like chapters in a textbook and then reacting to the assessment at the end is perhaps the best way to describe it.

In this way, our soul learns and continues to the next challenge, the next teaching tool, seeing each to broaden and expand our learning and our ability to learn. Perhaps today's human progress from one academic test to another, each based on what we have just been taught. We lose track of the way life teaches us and teaches our soul. Tests for our soul are cumulative; the events and

---

[190] Ibid.
[191] Wikipedia, "Lucy Australopithecus."
[192] "Extinction."

challenges may be discreet, but once we have passed through each one, what we have learned becomes a part of our makeup, which, collectively, I applied to the next challenge.

The reincarnated soul is interested in progress to the last visit to the physical realm, the ultimate challenges, the final karmic learning, in order to ascend to the higher realm. It can develop and change, as are physical beings, able to develop and adapt to the changing life forces, just as Darwin's finches have.

Our interconnection means the spiritual knowledge we gain through each lifetime benefits not only you, individually, but humanity in the complete picture.

Your intrinsic reason for incarnating gradually becomes easier and easier to discern. You discover you are here to be of service. Eventually, you reach a level of development where you serve as a teacher or guide for other souls. This is sometimes referred to as "Ascension."[193]
There are no signposts to the essential meaning of what it is we have to learn in this crucible of life's challenges. I recall my parents discussing forms my friend's parents were asking mine to countersign. Compared to the issues of their son's hearing impairment, completing forms and getting someone to countersign them seemed soul-crushing, erroneous details, acting like fog, obscuring the real learning that is required. Yet those forms drew my parents into coming of the peripheral challenges his parents faced all the time.

So, no matter what choices you make in life, all is well because you are repeatedly given a further opportunity to learn. Each life event is a course in your earthly classroom that is set in motion by the soul agreements you've put in place. Your awareness of "why you are here now," will expand when you accept that what needs to happen simply happens. Or to put it slightly differently, when you accept that events and people in your life are put in place to enhance the evolution of your soul and that of others, then you know that such life lessons stem from the wisdom of your soul and your guides' prodding. [194]

Every lifetime has a soul-designed curriculum for enhancing and expanding your soul awareness and capability. Certain past lives result in your freewill missteps that leave you with karma. Other past lives are ones of accomplishing your soul intentions, bringing about dharma. When you accept that all experiences in life serve the purpose of moving to a higher "grade" in the school of soul development, life becomes manageable. All the events in your life offer you the window to know who you are, why you are here, and how you can continue to advance as a soul. Benevolent spiritual guidance is available to you, always to support your onward journey. The very best advice I can offer is to trust and accept fear as a signal that you are facing an opening to grow. [195]

As our soul moves from one life to another collecting good and bad Karma, we will be presented knowing that it will help us navigate through the challenges of this physical life. We will accumulate new karmic trends, some good and some bad, resolve past events and outcomes from challenges.

Yes. We can record the demise of species of animals within a collective human lifetime. Through evolution, species arise through the process of speciation—where new varieties of organisms arise

---

[193] https://www.ravenheartcenter.com/index.php/soul-evolution, "Soul Evolution Clear Past Life Karma and Live Your Life Purpose."
[194] Ibid.
[195] Ibid.

and thrive when they can find and exploit an ecological niche—and species become extinct when they can no longer survive in changing conditions or against superior competition. The relationship between animals and their ecological niches has been firmly established. A typical species becomes extinct within 10 million years of its first appearance, although some species, called living fossils, survive with little to no morphological change for hundreds of millions of years.[196]

A soul incarnated several hundred years ago would face dramatically different social and physical challenges and outcomes from today or a hundred years in the future. But all challenges and outcomes are consistent with the time in which the incarnation took place.

---

[196] Wikipedia, "Extinction."

## 34   Differing Pace of Evolution and Karma

T he argument that Darwinian evolution, and the interconnected nature of environmental changes, affecting plants, animals, and humans, move at such a slow pace that its impact on souls being reincarnated into living beings is marginal. It is working on a different time frame. It is shorter than the time scale of the universe from the Big Bang. Detailed measurements of the expansion rate of the universe place the Big Bang at around 13.8 billion years ago, which is thus considered the age of the universe.[197]

While shamans appeared in the Paleolithic. The Paleolithic, also called the Old Stone Age, is a period in human prehistory distinguished by the original development of stone tools that cover c. 99% of the time of human technological prehistory. It extends from the earliest known use of stone tools by hominids c. 3.3 million years ago, to the end of the Pleistocene c. 11,650 cal BP.[198]

Both use the same time scale, a year, but one is described in Billions, while the other is measured in millions.

If you had been a soul incarnated into a cave dweller in the Paleolithic, your ability to learn, the challenges and opportunities would have been consistent with what you experienced. There is no limit on what it is a soul needs to learn in order to ascend to a level where incarnation no longer occurs. You have become an ascended being.

We look at Lucy and her world, how she lived life and the community she was in, as best we can through the archaeological record. From this information, we try to infer the life she led. The soul in her when she passed over will have reincarnated many, many times since then. It will carry with it experiences and teachings from her into each subsequent incarnation. It will learn and develop as all creatures do, but the pace will differ from the Darwinian record.

The underlying archaeological record, and the evidence Darwin noted for species selection and adaptation, need to be slower, must be slower than the spiritual changes the soul will undergo in each lifetime. Evolution of the soul is not a linear progression; different things need to be learned in each period of physical existence.

A shaman may help a soul reincarnate, but they cannot influence the nature of karmic reincarnation. The shaman cannot affect the karmic history of the soul at the point of reincarnation. Karmically, if a soul must repeat a certain challenge, the shaman cannot influence that, just as they cannot influence when that repetition may occur.

A soul experiencing the challenge of deafness in the 16th century may incarnate with deafness as a renewed challenge in the 21st century because what was karmically learned in the past either needs refinement only the 21st century can provide, or, there is more to learn.

The soul develops because of its experiences; it develops at the pace those experiences are presented to it. Karma is not a judge of what experiences are presented, or when or in what guise they offered. It does not determine what must be learned in the physical world's existence. Karma is not one enormous challenge that must be learned from; it is about all the soul's existence.

---

[197] "Big Bang."
[198] "Paleolithic."

A soul may be challenged to compassionately support and help a wife, child, friend, or family member that is experiencing a physical or emotional disability. And yet Karma will consider how the soul interacts with the assistant at the burger restaurant drive thru.

## 35 Bibliography

Bibliography:

Britannica. "Bardo ThöDol Tibetan Buddhist Text."

Collection, University of California Press eBook. "The Spiritual Quest." (1982–2004).

Dharmakaya. "Dharmakaya Buddhist Concept."

Dictionary, Merriam-Webster. "Definition of Soul by Merriam-Webster."

GotQuestions.org. "What is the difference between the Soul and Spirit of Man?"

http://healerofheartsandminds.com. "Reincarnation, Past Lives, Suffering and the Bible, a Shaman's Views."

http://vajranatha.com. "Ancient Tibetan Bonpo Shamanism."

http://veda.wikidot.com/karma. "Karma Veda."

https://carljungdepthpsychologysite.blog/2019/04/29/carl-jung-on-the-tibetan-book-of-the-dead/#.Xmt2-qrX23A. "Carl Jung on the Tibetan Book of the Dead–Carl Jung Depth Psychology."

https://en.wikipedia.org/wiki/Charles_Darwin. "Charles Darwin."

https://en.wikipedia.org/wiki/Karma. "Karma."

https://en.wikipedia.org/wiki/Neuroplasticity. "Neuroplasticity."

https://en.wikipedia.org/wiki/The_City_of_God. "The City of God."

https://evolution.berkeley.edu/evolibrary/article/evo_14. "Mechanisms the Processes of Evolution."

https://glyndwr.repository.guildhe.ac.uk/246/1/fulltext.pdf. "Jung and World Religions."

https://learningenglish.voanews.com/a/a-new-reason-for-why-the-deaf-may-have-trouble-reading-119728279/115194.html. "A New Reason Why the Deaf May Have Trouble Reading."

https://link.springer.com/article/10.1186/s40613-015-0016-2. "On the Naturalization of Karma and Rebirth."

https://news.harvard.edu/gazette/story/2006/02/meditation-found-to-increase-brain-size/. "Meditation Found to Increase Brain Size."

https://news.harvard.edu/gazette/story/2010/11/wandering-mind-not-a-happy-mind/. "Wandering Mind Not a Happy Mind."

https://os.me/four-types-of-karma-explained-understanding-karma/. "4 Types of Karma–Understanding Karma in Spirituality."

https://www.allaboutsikhs.com/sikhism-faqs/sikhism-faqswhat-is-karma. "Sikhism FAQs What Is Karma?"

https://www.britannica.com/science/cross-modal-plasticity. "Cross-Modal Plasticity Biology Britannica."

https://www.budsas.org/ebud/whatbudbeliev/96.htm. "What Buddhists Believe–Rebirth."

https://www.disabilityexpertsfl.com/blog/difficulties-the-deaf-face-every-day. "Difficulties the Hearing Impaired Face Every Day."

https://www.hinduwebsite.com/hinduism/h_karma.asp. "What Is Karma in Hinduism?"

https://www.infoplease.com/us/major-religions-world/hinduism. "Hinduism."

https://www.merriam-webster.com/dictionary/symbiotic. "Definition of Symbiotic."

https://www.ncregister.com/blog/robert-barron/grace-or-karma. "Grace or Karma."

https://www.physicsclassroom.com/class/newtlaws/Lesson-4/Newton-s-Third-Law. "Newton's Third Law of Motion."

https://www.ravenheartcenter.com/index.php/soul-evolution. "Soul Evolution Clears Past Life Karma and Live Your Life Purpose."

https://www.sciencedirect.com/topics/medicine-and-dentistry/neural-plasticity. "Neural Plasticity."

https://www.signia-hearing.com/blog/how-does-hearing-loss-affect-the-brain/. "How Hearing Loss Affects the Brain and Associated Risks—Signia Hearing Aids."

https://www.taosnews.com/stories/ancient-wisdom-of-the-himalayas, 60208. "Ancient Wisdom of the Himalayas."

https://www.wisdomlib.org. "Antarabhava, AntarāBhava 2 Definitions."

International, Ligmincha. "Message from Dalai Lama.Pdf."

jainbelief.com. "Jainism."

Lionsroar.com. "The Four Points of Letting Go in the Bardo."

Merriam-Webster. "Definition of New Age."

Mirror, the. "'The Tibetan Book of the Dead' and Vajrayana."

Philosophy, Stanford Encyclopedia of. "Descartes and the Pineal Gland."

Pratt, David. "Fate or Free Will?"

Wikipedia. "History of the Location of the Soul."

Wikipedia. "Alfred Russel Wallace."

———. "Artha."

———. "Ascended Master."

———. "Atheism."

———. "Atman."

———. "Balarama."

———. "Bardo."

———. "Bardo Thodol."

———. "Bhagavad Gita."

———. "Big Bang."

———. "Buddhism."

———. "Carl Jung."

———. "Catholic Church."

———. "Causality."

———. "Caveman."

———. "Coevolution."

———. "Darwinism."

———. "Dharma."

———. "Extinction."

———. "Hinduism."

———. "History of Hearing Aids."

———. "Isaac Newton."

———. "Jainism."

———. "Jarasandha."

———. "John Burroughs."

———. "Kama."

———. "Karma in Tibetan Buddhism."

———. "Krishna."

———. "Kriyamana Karma."

———. "Lucy Australopithecus."

———. "Mahabharata."

———. "Moksha."

———. "Monotheism."

———. "Muslims."

———. "Paleolithic."
———. "Pandava."
———. "Phala."
———. "Polytheism."
———. "Protestantism."
———. "PuruṣāRtha."
———. "Religion in Tibet."
———. "Richard Dawkins."
———. "Robert Thurman."
———. "Samskara."
———. "Sanchita Karma."
———. "Sikhism."
———. "Skandha."
———. "Soul."
———. "Tahrif."
———. "Taoism."
———. "Tawhid."
———. "Three marks of Existence."
———. "Tibetan Buddhism."
———. "Vajrasattva."
———. "Vedas."
Woolger, Dr. Roger J. "Beyond Death—Transition and the Afterlife."
www.rigpawiki.org. "Emptiness."
———. "Nyingma Buddhism."